Contents

About the authors

Mark Greener spent a decade in biomedical research before joining *MIMS Magazine* for GPs in 1989. Since then, he has written on health and biology for magazines worldwide for non-specialists, healthcare professionals and scientists. He is the author of 12 other books, including *Coping with Asthma in Adults* (2011) and *The Heart Attack Survival Guide* (2012), both Sheldon Press. Mark lives with his wife, three children and two cats in a Cambridgeshire village.

Christine Craggs-Hinton, mother of three, followed a career in the civil service until, in 1991, she developed fibromyalgia, a chronic pain condition. Christine took up writing for therapeutic reasons, and has in the past few years produced more than a dozen books for Sheldon Press, including *Living with Fibromyalgia*, *The Chronic Fatigue Healing Diet*, *Coping Successfully with Psoriasis* and *How to Lower Your Blood Pressure*. Since moving to the Canary Islands, where she is the resident agony aunt for a local paper, she has also taken up fiction writing.

Introduction

A century ago, children with diabetes lived on death row. Most slipped into a fatal coma within a few months of developing the disease.[1,2] Since then, doctors and scientists have made remarkable progress in understanding and treating diabetes. Nevertheless, it still causes around 1 in 8 deaths among people aged 20 to 79 years in the UK, according to Diabetes UK. Indeed, poorly controlled diabetes can cut up to 20 years from your life expectancy. And it's on the rise. Every 3 or 4 minutes someone, somewhere in the UK receives the life-changing news that they have developed diabetes. Indeed, around 1 person in every 20 in the UK has diabetes – that's around 2.9 million people in 2011. To make matters even worse, up to half a million people in the UK have undiagnosed diabetes. The first hint may be a serious complication such as poor vision, a heart attack or impotence. Indeed, half of people with type 2 diabetes mellitus (T2DM) – the type that usually, but not always, emerges in middle age – develop complications before their doctor diagnoses diabetes.

Tragically, much of this suffering could be avoided if people took control of their diabetes sooner. This book shows how a healthy, balanced diet helps avoid the worse ravages of diabetes. In some people with the early stages of the most common form of diabetes, a healthy diet and lifestyle can reverse the apparently inexorable decline. Unfortunately, diet and lifestyle changes alone usually cannot prevent diabetes-related damage to our critical organs. Many people with diabetes also need to take antidiabetic drugs or inject insulin. Yet even in people taking the most modern medicines, following a healthy, balanced diet still increases their chances of avoiding diabetes-related damage, disability and even premature death.

A complex disease with a simple cause

Diabetes is a complex disease with a simple cause. Cells are, essentially, biological factories. And all factories need fuel. Cells use a type of sugar called glucose to power their activities. The body extracts glucose from the carbohydrates (such as sugars and starch) that we consume as part of our daily diet.

Maintaining adequate levels of glucose in the blood is essential for survival. But people with diabetes have too much of a good thing. Their dangerously high blood sugar levels poison their cells. As a result, poorly treated diabetes can cause debilitating, distressing and disabling complications such as pain, ulcers, amputations, heart disease and blindness. So, treating diabetes aims to control blood glucose levels and counter other factors that worsen the prospects for people with diabetes, such as smoking, obesity and raised concentrations of cholesterol.

Changing diet is one of the longest established treatments for raised blood sugar levels. The Hindu physician Sushruta, probably writing around the sixth century BCE, noted that the urine of people with diabetes attracted ants (the sugar in the urine appealed to the insects). Sushruta suggested exercise and vegetables for corpulent people with diabetes and a nourishing diet for lean patients, who he rightly recognized had a more severe form of the disease.[3]

Sushruta's insights were remarkably prescient. But doctors' view of the ideal diet for people with diabetes has changed dramatically over the decades. For example, in the years just before the first successful treatment with insulin in 1922, some doctors told patients to eat large amounts of fat – the reverse of advice today – and cut back on carbohydrate.[1,2] Around the same time, some doctors suggested diets for people with diabetes based around specific foods, including skimmed milk, potatoes and oatmeal.[3]

Other doctors, led by Frederick Madison Allen, suggested cutting carbohydrate consumption dramatically, often to starvation levels. People with diabetes following the Allen diet ate a maximum of 600 ml of clear meat soup and between three and six bran muffins daily for 10 days. They then gradually increased their carbohydrate intake until the doctor detected sugars in their urine. Patients kept their carbohydrate intake below this level. Cooks even boiled vegetables three times to remove as much carbohydrate as possible.[1,2,3] Of course, this also removed many valuable nutrients.

One of these patients, Elizabeth Hughes, the 11-year-old diabetic daughter of an American presidential candidate and New York Governor, controlled her blood sugar levels by eating just 500 to 800 calories a day. She also fasted for 1 day a week. If doctors detected even a trace of sugar in her urine she ate 250 calories a day or less. Her weight fell from 34 kg in 1919 (average for her age and height) to 20 kg in the summer of 1922. Fortunately, in the August of that year Elizabeth was among the first people treated with insulin. Elizabeth recovered, travelling widely and working with numerous charities. She died in 1981.[1,2]

As we will see during this book, a healthy, balanced diet remains a foundation of diabetic care, almost a century after insulin's introduction. Watching your diet helps control blood glucose levels and so can reduce the risk of complications. But, ironically, unhealthy, unbalanced diets also contribute to most cases of diabetes.

The dangers of a poor diet

Humans did not evolve to chomp on junk food high in sugar and fat, and low in essential nutrients: sweets, cakes, takeaway food, ready meals and so on. We evolved to eat, essentially, a hunter–gatherer diet – one that is rich in complex carbohydrates (such as starch from fruit and vegetables) and low in animal fats. Our hunter–gatherer ancestors also kept moving searching for food and water. Inevitably, most members of these societies were physically fit and relatively lean.

By contrast, the typical modern Western diet produces an overabundance of energy. If you do not burn this energy off, the body stores the surplus in fat cells as a precaution against famine. But in industrialized nations we can easily access food. So, we never use these stores. As a result we gain weight, especially around the middle (central obesity). This excess weight causes around 90 per cent of cases of T2DM in the UK. Obesity also increases the risk of stroke, heart disease and some cancers.

Excess weight is not the only cause of diabetes. For example, diabetes can arise from 'biological civil war' when the body mistakenly destroys insulin-producing cells. And certain medicines, operations, diseases and even pregnancy can trigger diabetes.

Nevertheless, our expanding waistbands are responsible for most of the rise in diabetes that experts expect will emerge over the next few years. The upward trend is already clear: according to government statistics, the number of drugs prescribed for diabetes in England increased by 41 per cent between 2005/6 and 2010/11. And while the number of new cases diagnosed each year is already frightening, it will probably get worse. In 2008, doctors diagnosed 145,000 new cases of diabetes, which Diabetes UK points out is more than the population of Middlesbrough. Diabetes UK also predicts that by 2025, 4.2 million people will have diabetes, up from 2.6 million in 2009. Meanwhile, increasing numbers of overweight and obese children and adolescents will develop T2DM.

Now the good news

Now some good news. Healthy eating – alongside other lifestyle changes and, if necessary, drugs – dramatically reduces the risk of diabetic complications. If you are already taking insulin or antidiabetic tablets, diet alone will not control your blood glucose levels. Nevertheless, eating a healthy, balanced diet will reduce the risk of complications, both long-term (e.g. heart disease, amputations and blindness) and short-term (e.g. hypoglycaemic attacks caused by dangerously low blood sugar levels). Indeed, a healthy diet helps people with diabetes live fulfilled, active, satisfying lives.

If you've not yet developed full-blown T2DM, but are at risk – so-called prediabetes or impaired glucose tolerance – improving your eating habits can go a long way towards slowing the progression to diabetes and, in some cases, may reverse the gradual increase in blood glucose levels that ends in your doctor diagnosing diabetes. So, if T2DM runs in your family, your doctor has diagnosed prediabetes, or you are overweight and inactive, you should try hard to eat a healthy diet, exercise, quit smoking and follow the other suggestions in this book. A healthy diet and lifestyle will also help reduce your risk of developing many other serious diseases.

This book begins by looking at the causes and consequences of diabetes. We will consider the place of diet in diabetes management, alongside other treatments. Unlike a century ago, doctors now suggest that most people with diabetes can choose from a wide range of foods. With some planning you should be able to find a healthy diet that reduces your risk of diabetes-related complications, while satisfying your taste buds. We wish you all the best in your endeavours to eat yourself back to much better health and peace of mind.

Authors' note to the reader

This book aims to help you improve your control of blood glucose levels, avoid short- and long-term complications, and enhance your general health and well-being. The NHS now recommends that everyone with diabetes should take part in 'structured education' to help manage his or her disease. These courses cover lifestyle changes (including diet), medications and monitoring blood glucose. For example, DAFNE (Dose Adjustment For Normal Eating) and DESMOND (Diabetes Education and Self-Management for Ongoing and Newly Diagnosed diabetes) help people with types 1 and 2 diabetes, respectively. If you want to know more or want a refresher, speak to your GP or diabetes team. The advice in this book supports and expands on, rather than replaces, these self-management courses and suggestions from your healthcare professionals, which are tailored to your particular problems and circumstances.

If you think you are at risk of diabetes or you develop symptoms (see page 21) you must see your GP as soon as possible. Finally, although changing your diet can help improve your blood glucose levels you should never adjust or stop any medicine (for diabetes or any other disease) without speaking to your doctor or diabetes nurse first.

1

The pancreas – controlling glucose levels

Diagnosing disease has never been easy. Medieval doctors regularly inspected their patients' urine by holding a sample in a bulbous glass flask to the light. Some went further: they took a swig. Indian texts from the fifth century BCE and the Islamic philosopher–scientist Avicenna, writing around the start of the eleventh century, commented that the urine of people with diabetes tasted sweet. In 1674, Thomas Willis, a leading English doctor, used the sweet taste to distinguish diabetes from other diseases that caused frequent urination, such as infections or bladder stones. Willis coined the term diabetes mellitus – the latter term from the Greek word for honey or sweet.[1]

As mentioned in the introduction, cells use glucose for fuel. Glucose is the most common sugar in the human body. Carbohydrates are long chains of sugars; starch, for example, consists of long chains of glucose. Sucrose (table sugar) contains glucose joined to another sugar called fructose. Digestion breaks carbohydrates into single sugars, which travel around your body in your blood.

A hormone called insulin stimulates cells to take glucose from the blood. Cells then use the glucose to generate energy. Without insulin, most cells (there are some important exceptions) cannot use glucose so, in people who do not produce enough insulin, glucose levels in the blood rise. In other people with diabetes, insulin does not work properly when it reaches the cells – so-called insulin resistance (some people have both problems). Again, the cells do not absorb glucose and the amount in the blood (the concentration) rises.

In response, the body tries to flush the excess sugar out of the body. As a result, people with diabetes urinate more – and their urine tastes sweet. Diabetes derives from another Greek word that means siphon. The second century Greek doctor Aretus the Cappadocian described patients passing urine 'like a siphon'.[1]

To understand what goes wrong in diabetes and why a healthy, balanced diet helps, we need to look at how the body normally controls blood sugar levels. In this chapter we will discuss the pancreas, insulin's actions and how the body tightly regulates blood glucose levels. Some of this section may seem a little complicated at first. But it is important to understand the basic principles of glucose control. So take your time, and, if need be, discuss individual points further with your doctor, nurse or a helpline such as that run by Diabetes UK. See the list of useful addresses, beginning on page 121, for the contact details of all the organizations mentioned in this book.

The pancreas

The pancreas, which is about 15 cm (6 inches) long, lies behind your stomach about level with the inverted V where your ribs meet at the front of your chest (see Figure 1). The rounded 'head' of the pancreas is next to the first part of your bowel after your stomach – called the duodenum. Biologists distinguish two other parts of the pancreas: the middle 'body' and the narrow 'tail', which lies on the left side of your body (Figure 2).

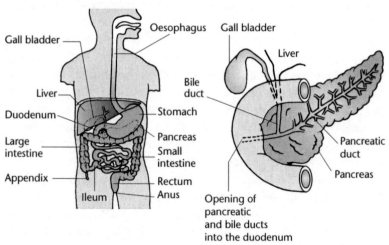

Figure 1 The digestive system   **Figure 2 The pancreas**

Your pancreas has two vital roles, producing:

- pancreatic juice, a cocktail of chemicals that helps you digest food, and
- several important hormones, including insulin.

Pancreatic juice

When you eat, food travels from your mouth, down your oesophagus and into your stomach. Acid produced by the stomach sterilizes, and starts digesting, food. From the stomach, food flows into the duodenum (see Figure 1).

Specialist cells in the pancreas (acinar cells) pump pancreatic juice into small ducts. These tubes feed into a larger duct running the length of the organ – the pancreatic duct (see Figure 2). Meanwhile, the liver and gall bladder (a small pouch under the liver) release a greenish-yellow fluid called bile, which helps digest fats. The gall bladder stores bile made earlier. Bile flows along ducts from the liver and gall bladder, which join to form the common bile duct and enter the head of the pancreas. The common bile duct and pancreatic duct converge, then join the duodenum.

The composition of pancreatic juice

Pancreatic juice contains:

- water;
- enzymes that digest proteins (proteases), fat (pancreatic lipase) starch (amylase) and several other constituents of food;
- bicarbonate to neutralize the acid that arrives in the small intestine from the stomach. Cells lining the pancreatic duct add the bicarbonate, which acts as a natural antacid.

Islands in a pancreatic sea

Doctors recognized millennia ago that the urine of people with diabetes tasted sweet. However, the cause of the sweet taste remained a mystery. Nineteenth-century doctors discovered that many people who died from diabetes had damaged pancreases. Then, between 1867 and 1869, a German medical student called Paul Langerhans scrutinized the pancreas under a microscope. In a 'sea' of acinar cells, Langerhans saw small, pale 'islands'. But doctors still did not know what these 'Islets of Langerhans' did.[2]

Another piece of the jigsaw fell into place in 1889, when German researchers found that if they surgically removed a dog's pancreas, the unfortunate canine developed diabetes. However, when they tied the pancreatic duct, the dog experienced minor digestive problems but not diabetes. So, researchers realized that the pancreas controlled blood sugar levels.

We now know that the Islets of Langerhans produce hormones, including insulin and glucagon, which work together to maintain the proper level of sugar in the blood. Each of the million or so islets contain three major types of cell:

- Beta cells produce insulin and make up about 60–80 per cent of the islets. The term insulin comes from the Latin for island: insula.
- Alpha cells produce glucagon, which essentially has the opposite actions to insulin.
- Delta cells secrete the hormone somatostatin. This, in turn, controls the release of other hormones, including glucagon.

Pancreatic islets also produce several minor hormones. We won't consider somatostatin or these other hormones any further.

Cells from your big toe to your scalp need insulin to ensure they generate sufficient energy to survive. So, a dense network of blood vessels carries hormones secreted by the pancreas around the body. Indeed, while the Islets of Langerhans account for about 1–2 per cent of the weight of the pancreas, they receive around 10–15 per cent of the organ's blood flow.

Insulin

Insulin is one of the most important hormones released by the pancreas. It's so important that evolution ensured the protein differs little between mammals (see box opposite). Even dung beetles produce insulin. So why is insulin so important?

Proteins, amino acids and insulin

When you eat meat or another protein, your digestive system breaks protein into its building blocks – called amino acids. Humans use 20 different amino acids to build proteins as varied as the muscles in your heart, the nerves in your brain and the hairs on your head. The sequence of amino acids determines the size, shape and function of each protein.

Your body rearranges the amino acids in food into the proteins that your body needs. That's why you can convert a steak into your hair, nails, skin, blood and so on. Our bodies can make only about half of the 20 amino acids we need. We need to get the rest – the so-called essential amino acids – from food. Think of a protein as a tower of Lego bricks. Digestion pulls the tower apart into separate bricks. Your body rejoins the bricks to form a new tower with a different order, shape and size.

Insulin contains 51 amino acids (the bricks). Cow (bovine) insulin differs by three amino acids and pig (porcine) insulin by just one. The resemblance is so close that people with diabetes can control blood sugar levels by injecting insulin extracted from pigs, cows and even fish. A once widely used insulin contained 70 per cent beef insulin and 30 per cent pork insulin, for example. Nevertheless, pharmaceutical companies needed to process 8000 lbs of animal pancreases to extract 1 lb of insulin (3,600 kg to produce 1 kg).

Over the years, animal insulin saved countless lives. Today, people with diabetes tend to use genetically engineered insulin that exactly reproduces the human sequence. This is available in almost unlimited amounts and avoids any potential infections and other risks (such as triggering immune reactions) associated with proteins derived from animals. We'll look at therapeutic insulin again in Chapter 5.

Glucose from food

Next time you pick up a potato look at all that white flesh inside the skin. The potato plant stores energy as starch in the flesh, which it uses to support growth. And that's why potatoes became a staple food worldwide: they are packed with energy and nutrients. Indeed, we obtain most of our daily glucose from starchy carbohydrates such as rice, pasta, potatoes and bread as well as from the sugars in, for example, fruit and sweet foods. Digestion breaks starch and sugars into glucose. So, after we eat, blood glucose levels rise. But to what extent and for how long depends on whether we ate a baked potato or drank a bottle of sugary soft drink.

Blood glucose levels shoot up within a few minutes of swallowing a sugary drink. Some people find this provides a short-lived lift. However, they then report feeling a little tired and maybe a bit downcast as blood sugar levels fall. The body takes longer to convert starchy carbohydrates (such as in the baked potato) into sugars. This slow release of glucose helps smooth out the peaks and troughs in blood sugar. That's good news for everyone; it helps stop you snacking between meals and so controls weight, for example. And it helps people with diabetes avoid potentially dangerous declines in their blood sugar level – hypoglycaemic attacks (see page 38).

After you eat...

Your cells need glucose all day, not just after you eat. So, you have various stores around your body. Before a meal, your liver and, to a lesser extent, kidneys release glucose from their stores. When you wake in the morning, your liver has produced about 80 per cent of the glucose in your blood. Your kidneys have released the other 20 per cent. Indeed, when insulin levels are low, production of glucose from your liver and kidney can double.[3]

After a meal, levels of glucose in the blood rise rapidly, triggering beta cells to release insulin. In response, the amount of glucose released from the liver declines by almost 80 per cent. The sight and taste of food can also trigger insulin release, which helps your body prepare for the expected surge in glucose after a meal. Several other food molecules, such as amino acids and fats, can also stimulate insulin release.

Measuring blood glucose levels

Doctors can report blood glucose levels using several different units. In the UK, doctors usually use millimoles of glucose per litre of blood (mmol/l). Clinicians in the USA typically use milligrams (mg) of glucose per 100 ml (dl) of blood. A blood sugar level of 80 mg/dl is around 4.4 mmol/l. To convert mg/dl to mmol/l, multiply by 0.0555. To convert mmol/l to mg/dl, multiply by 18.0182.

Before a meal, the fasting blood glucose concentration (12–16 hours after you last ate) in a healthy person is around 4.4–5.0 mmol/l. At these levels of glucose, insulin secretion is very low. Blood glucose levels peak between 60 and 90 minutes after eating a meal and can reach around 9 mmol/l. Insulin secretion rises in parallel with the increasing blood glucose levels.

In healthy people blood glucose levels return to premeal concentrations after around 3 hours, and insulin secretion drops. Nevertheless, insulin controls sugar levels throughout the day. So, only about half the insulin released by the pancreas follows the spike in blood glucose levels after a meal. You slowly release the remaining insulin over the rest of the day.

Insulin's actions

Insulin stimulates cells to absorb enough glucose from the blood to make the energy needed to keep us alive and active. To do this, insulin binds to specific receptors on the surface of the muscle, fat and other cells.

When insulin binds to the receptor, special proteins called glucose transporters move from the inside of the cell to the membrane that surrounds each cell. The transporter picks up a molecule of glucose, which it carries to the inside of the cell. When blood levels of insulin fall, glucose transporters remain inside the cell waiting for the next meal. Meanwhile, cells switch to alternative energy sources, such as fat.

Some organs – of which the brain is the most important – do not store glucose, and its cells, unlike those of many other organs, can't effectively use fatty acids as a fuel (see below). So, the brain depends on a constant supply of glucose from your blood. And it's always hungry. Indeed, your brain uses around a quarter of all the glucose in your body.

So that the body can supply the brain and other vital organs with glucose during times of famine, insulin stimulates the liver to store some of the glucose in a meal. Most of the blood supply from your gut, which carries the nutrients you've ingested from your food, goes through the liver before reaching the rest of the body. Between 25 and 30 per cent of the glucose you absorbed from the food is removed from the blood on its way through the liver. The liver uses about 60 per cent of this glucose to fuel its activities and sticks the rest together into a long chain called glycogen. Muscles can also store glycogen, which holds the energy ready for future use – a bit like a biological battery.

The liver and muscle can store about 2,000 calories-worth of energy in a 70 kg person. A moderately active person needs about 35 calories a day for each kg of body weight to keep their weight stable. Sedentary people and those who exercise vigorously need about 29 and 40 calories, respectively, for each kg of body weight. In other words, glycogen stores are enough to keep an average woman going for a day.

The liver's storage capacity is limited. Once glycogen stores make up more than about 5 per cent of the weight of the liver, the body strongly suppresses glycogen production. But all that glucose in the diet is too valuable to waste. So, liver cells use the additional glucose to make fatty acids, which are released into the circulation and used by other tissues as a source of energy when there's not enough glucose.

To further bolster our energy reserves, insulin inhibits the breakdown of fat and encourages fat cells (adipocytes) to take up glucose. Fat cells use glucose to make another chemical called glycerol. Usually about 5 per cent of the glucose in a meal ends up as glycerol. Fat cells join glycerol with fatty acids to form a fat called triglyceride – yet another energy store. In a 70 kg adult the body stores around 100,000 calories as triglycerides, especially in layers of fat around the stomach. Unfortunately, high levels of triglycerides in the blood increase the risk of heart disease and pancreatitis (where the pancreas becomes inflamed [page 20]).

So many energy stores may seem superfluous – biological belt and braces – when we can just pop down to the supermarket. But people living in developed countries have been able to rely on secure food sources for a relatively short time. Previous generations endured times of feast and times of famine. The winters of even good years often proved tough. These diverse energy stores increased our ancestors' chances of survival when food was scarce.

Insulin has yet another action that helps us survive food shortages – to stimulate cells to take up amino acids. You can see its effects in people with anorexia – they seem little more than skin and bones. In particular they lack muscle. When insulin levels are low and we have depleted our other energy stores, cells start breaking down protein in our muscle. This releases amino acids into the bloodstream. The liver can convert some of these amino acids into glucose, a process called gluconeogenesis.

Glucagon: insulin's partner

Almost all biological actions have an opposite and equal reaction. This fundamental process (homeostasis) means that the vital biological mechanisms we rely on to remain healthy stay within relatively narrow limits.

For example, another hormone, glucagon, has the opposite effect to insulin and increases blood glucose levels. As blood levels of glucose rise, glucagon secretion declines. The interplay between insulin and glucagon determines and, in healthy people, tightly controls blood glucose concentrations. So, when blood glucose levels fall, glucagon secretion increases, which:

- triggers liver cells to break down glycogen stores, thus releasing glucose into the blood;
- activates gluconeogenesis, in which the liver converts other substances, such as certain amino acids, into glucose; and
- stimulates the breakdown of triglycerides into fatty acids. Most cells can use the released fatty acids as fuel, which helps conserve dwindling glucose levels for organs (such as the brain) that cannot use fatty acids.

Exercise also triggers glucagon release, at least in part because working out burns up glucose.

A healthy pancreas has around a million Islets of Langerhans. So, we can lose a relatively large proportion – often more than 90 per cent – of our beta cells before the pancreas produces insufficient insulin to control swings in blood glucose levels. Essentially, diabetes arises when insulin production is no longer adequate to tightly control blood glucose concentrations.

2

Types of diabetes and their symptoms

We often talk about diabetes as if it's two diseases – type 1 diabetes mellitus (T1DM), which usually starts in children, and T2DM, which typically emerges in overweight, middle-aged people. In fact, diabetes has at least 50 possible causes.[1] And while you've probably heard that diabetes starts with a raging thirst, there are a wide range of symptoms.

The many faces of diabetes

For hundreds of years, physicians recognized that children with diabetes tended to die within a few months, whereas older people experienced fewer problems, in the short-term at least.[2] But doctors only formally subdivided diabetes mellitus, the most common type, into two – T1DM and T2DM – in the 1930s.

Some doctors add a third type of diabetes mellitus, which seems to be linked to Alzheimer's disease. A similar process that damages the brain, leading to dementia, seems to destroy pancreatic cells, leading to diabetes. However, T3DM isn't well characterized and we won't consider it further.

Type 1 diabetes mellitus

Normally, our immune system specifically attacks invading pathogens (such as bacteria, viruses and parasites), while limiting 'collateral' damage to healthy tissues. The immune system launches this targeted attack using proteins called antibodies, which identify the invaders and trigger the reactions that destroy the pathogens. Occasionally, however, the immune system can produce antibodies against healthy tissues (autoantibodies, a process called autoimmunity). For example:

- Rheumatoid arthritis arises when the immune system produces autoantibodies that destroy joints.
- Multiple sclerosis follows autoantibodies' attack on the fatty sheath that surrounds nerve cells in the brain, a bit like the plastic insulation that surrounds electric wires. The fatty sheath allows nerves to conduct signals properly. So the attack on the sheath produces the debilitating symptoms of multiple sclerosis.

T1DM arises when the immune system produces autoantibodies (cytoplasmic islet cell antibodies in the jargon) that destroy beta cells in the pancreas over a few weeks.[3] This destruction means that the pancreas no longer produces insulin. So, people with T1DM need regular insulin injections to replace the missing hormone (see Chapter 5). Indeed, until recently doctors often called T1DM insulin-dependent diabetes. But it's a misnomer. As we'll see, many people with T2DM eventually need insulin to control their blood sugar levels.

T1DM – a common disease

T1DM, which accounts for 10–15 per cent of cases of diabetes, can develop at any age, and symptoms generally emerge over several days to a few weeks. The symptoms of T1DM are also much more dramatic than in T2DM, which can emerge so slowly and insidiously that some people don't realize they have developed diabetes until they start suffering complications. Doctors usually diagnose T1DM in patients between 10 and 14 years of age. Most cases of T1DM appear before the age of 40 years. As adults can develop this type of diabetes, another old name for T1DM, juvenile diabetes, is another misnomer. Around 1 in every 700–1,000 children develops the condition and around 25,000 people in the UK under the age of 25 years have T1DM.

Genetics and diabetes

Doctors don't fully understand why the body wages immunological war on the pancreas. There's undoubtedly a genetic element. You probably know that DNA contains your genetic code. If you could stretch the DNA in a human cell in a single line, the strand would be around 2 metres long. So, DNA is compressed into the famous double helix. Our genetic code includes around 25,000 genes, which instruct your cells to make the proteins that, for example, keep your hair and toenails growing, the lens in your eye clear, and transfer signals inside and between your cells. Genes normally come in pairs. You inherited one from your biological mother, the other from your father. Some genes are abnormal (mutated). Usually mutations don't produce any effect. But in other cases, the mutation changes the instruction given by the gene. This in turn alters the protein's structure and function. It's a bit like switching a letter so that you change a word's meaning.

In some instances, the changes cause or increase your likelihood of developing certain diseases, including some forms of diabetes. Genetic tests can reveal whether one of the six subtypes of maturity-onset diabetes of the young (page 20) causes a person's diabetes and whether their children have inherited the affected gene.[4] Genetic diseases can cause several other types of diabetes. But these are rare and we won't look at them further.

Basically, if genes accounted for all the risk of developing a disease, the identical twin of a person with that disease (who shares the same genetic code) would inevitably develop the same condition. If environmental factors alone caused the condition, the identical twin's risk of developing the disease would be the same as that in the general population. As Table 1 shows, neither genetic nor environmental factors account fully for the risk of developing either T1DM or T2DM: both seem to contribute.

Table 1 The approximate risk of developing T1DM and T2DM if a family member also suffers from the disease

Relation of person with diabetes	Risk of developing	
	T1DM	T2DM
Mother	2%	–
Father	8%	–
Either parent	–	15%
Both parents	Up to 30%	75%
Brother/sister	10%	–
Non-identical twin	15%	10%
Identical twin	40%	90%

Source: Diabetes UK. *Diabetes in the UK 2010: Key statistics on diabetes.* <http://www.diabetes.org.uk/Documents/Reports/Diabetes_in_the_UK_2010.pdf>

The mystery of T1DM

In T1DM, environmental factors seem to interact with a genetic predisposition to trigger the immune system to destroy beta cells in the pancreas. The environmental triggers are something of a mystery, although infections probably cause some cases. For example, children born to women who contract rubella (German measles) during pregnancy seem particularly prone to developing T1DM.[5] Mumps can cause pancreatitis (page 20) and, in turn, may trigger diabetes.[1] That's another good reason to vaccinate your children. One of the authors contracted both German measles and mumps as a child and can still recall, more than 40 years later, just how awful these diseases are.

But not every child who contracts mumps develops diabetes, which underscores the importance of the genetic predisposition. And not everyone with diabetes contracted the infections linked to T1DM; other factors must contribute. For example, some studies suggest a link between T1DM and introducing cow's milk relatively early in an infant's diet. So, a short duration of breastfeeding may also increase the risk.[6]

Yet another theory places the blame for T1DM on the relative cleanliness of modern life in industrialized nations. The fate of several types of white blood cells – which fight infections – depends on the hazards in the environment. The immune system adapts to deal with the threats it is likely to encounter. Bacterial infections and certain parasites can programme the immune system to produce a particular type of white blood cell. This allows the immune system to respond quickly the next time you encounter the pathogen.

During the twentieth century, improved sanitation, better nutrition and vaccinations reduced the risk of infections. This has left the white blood cells with, essentially, nothing to do. Put rather simply, some of these idling white cells start attacking healthy tissues, which causes autoimmune diseases such as T1DM. Some scientists suggest that a similar process could contribute to the marked rise in allergies such as asthma and hay fever in the last few decades.

Nevertheless, identifying the exact causes of T1DM remains an area of intense interest to researchers, especially as the number of children under 15 years of age with T1DM is growing by around 3 per cent each year.[5] In part, the rise may reflect the success of treatment. People with T1DM live longer today than even in their grandparents' generation. So, they are more likely to pass any genes predisposing to T1DM on to their children.[7] Yet despite dramatic improvements in care, life expectancy among people with T1DM remains more than 20 years shorter than in the general population, underscoring the importance of a healthy, balanced diet and lifestyle.

Type 2 diabetes mellitus

According to Diabetes UK, T2DM accounts for between 85 and 90 per cent of the 2.9 million cases of diabetes in the UK. T2DM usually occurs in obese and overweight people aged over 40 years. Children with T1DM are not usually overweight or obese. However, in South Asian and black people, T2DM typically appears from the age of 25 years. Indeed, in 2000 doctors diagnosed the first cases of T2DM in children – in overweight girls aged between 9 and 16 years of Pakistani, Indian or Arabic origin. Doctors diagnosed the first cases in white children in 2002. Diabetes UK now estimates that up to 1,400 children in the UK have T2DM. T2DM has replaced the terms adult-onset diabetes, obesity-related diabetes and non-insulin-dependent diabetes.

The most common form of diabetes

The risk of developing diabetes rises sharply with advancing age, largely because T2DM becomes more common as people get older. In England in 2006, fewer than 1 in 100 men and women aged 16–24 years had diabetes. Among people aged 45–54 years rates were 6 per cent of men and almost 4 per cent of women. The proportions increased further to around 14 per cent of men and 11 per cent of women aged 75 years and above, Diabetes UK comments. Rates have probably risen since then.

Excess weight causes about 9 in every 10 cases of T2DM. However, understanding risk factors doesn't explain *what* goes wrong. Biologists now realize that three key changes underlie T2DM. The relative importance of each differs from person to person and doctors don't yet know which comes first:

- low production of insulin
- insulin resistance
- abnormalities in a group of hormones called incretins (see below).

Most people with T2DM show all three to a greater or lesser extent. And all three are progressive. That's why T2DM gradually gets worse, often despite medicines.

Low insulin production

People with T2DM still have some beta cells in their pancreas but these don't work properly. In the early stages of T2DM people do not secrete enough insulin to cope with the dramatic rise in glucose levels after a meal (technically called the postprandial level). The low insulin levels also mean that the liver doesn't reduce glucose production properly, which contributes to high postprandial blood sugar levels (Chapter 1).

As T2DM progresses, the amount of insulin produced by the pancreas declines as beta cells become less effective. So, levels of blood glucose gradually rise, even between meals. This worsening generally takes several years. By the time they are diagnosed, people with T2DM have typically lost between 50 and 70 per cent of their beta cell function.[8]

Insulin resistance

As T2DM progresses, muscle, liver, fat and other types of cell gradually respond less and less well to insulin. These insulin-resistant cells take up less glucose from the blood. In the early stages of T2DM, the pancreas produces more insulin to overcome the resistance. This increased production seems to be one of several factors that damage the pancreas, alongside fat deposits in beta cells and poisoning by high levels of glucose. Eventually, damaged beta cells can't produce sufficient insulin to overcome the resistance.[8]

Incretin abnormalities

Finally, a group of hormones produced in the gut – incretins – stops working properly. When doctors compared insulin production after patients took a certain amount of glucose by mouth and the same amount injected into the bloodstream they noticed something amiss. Glucose by mouth triggered much more insulin release than the same amount injected into the blood. In other words, the direct actions on the pancreas produced by glucose in the blood only partly account for insulin release.[8]

Further research revealed that glucose in food triggers the release of incretins by the gut. In turn, these hormones increase insulin secretion. This allows the body to prepare for the surge in glucose after a meal. Indeed, incretins account for up to half the production of insulin after a meal. Patients with T2DM lose around a quarter of their incretin function before they are diagnosed.[8] We'll return to incretins when we look at drugs used to treat T2DM (Chapter 5).

Incretins

Humans produce two main incretins called:

- GIP – glucose-dependent insulinotropic peptide; also known as gastric inhibitory peptide
- GLP-1 – glucagon-like peptide-1.

The natural history of type 2 diabetes

T2DM usually develops over many years, so there's a grey area between normal blood glucose levels and the concentrations doctors use to diagnose diabetes. Around seven million people in the UK are in this prediabetic grey zone.

Doctors use two diagnostic tests to detect prediabetes. An abnormal result on either suggests that your body isn't controlling glucose levels properly:

- Impaired fasting glucose (IFG; also called impaired fasting gly-caemia) measures your blood sugar level after you've not eaten ('fasted') overnight. A person with IFG shows a blood glucose concentration of at least 6.1 mmol/l but below 7.0 mmol/l. A level above 7.0 mmol/l probably means you have already developed diabetes. IFG also seems to indicate that you're more likely to develop heart disease or have a stroke. However, measuring fasting blood glucose can miss 20–30 per cent of cases of T2DM.

- Impaired glucose tolerance (IGT): Your doctor will ask you not to eat anything for 8–10 hours and then measure your blood glucose level. You'll then swallow a drink containing a known amount of glucose. Two hours later, the doctor takes another blood sample. People with IGT show glucose levels between 7.8 mmol/l and 11.1 mmol/l in this second sample.

Measuring blood glucose levels 2 hours after eating (the postprandial concentration) assesses your risk of developing serious problems more accurately than measuring fasting levels. For example, a study called DECODE showed that 33 per cent of men and 44 per cent of women had blood glucose levels that indicated diabetes 2 hours after eating, but were normal according to the fasting measurement. Patients with raised 2-hour blood glucose levels were 50 per cent more likely to die from cardiovascular disease and 100 per cent more likely to die from any cause during the study, which lasted on average almost 9 years, than people with normal blood glucose before and after eating.[9]

Prediabetes doesn't usually cause symptoms. Yet raised blood glucose levels, even below the threshold typically used to diagnose diabetes, can still damage your body. For example, about 8 per cent of people with IGT and 13 per cent of those with early diabetes already show damage to the delicate, light-sensitive layer at the back of their eyes (retinopathy; see page 51).[10]

So, as the name suggests, prediabetes means that you are well on the way to developing full-blown T2DM. On average, the risk of developing diabetes if you have normal blood glucose levels (normoglycaemia) is 0.7 per cent a year. In other words, each year fewer than 1 in 100 people with normal blood glucose levels develop T2DM. The risk rises to between 5 and 10 per cent in people with abnormal IFG or IGT.[10] However, this progression takes many years, influenced by a number of factors including:

- the severity of insulin resistance
- the extent of the decline in insulin production
- your age
- whether you have a family history of T2DM
- whether you're overweight or obese
- whether you previously developed diabetes during pregnancy (page 19).

This long delay between the start of prediabetes and the emergence of T2DM means you have plenty of time for a healthy, balanced diet and other lifestyle changes to make a difference. So, if you have any of the risk factors, such as obesity or other elements of the metabolic syndrome discussed in Chapter 3, it's probably worth asking your doctor to test to see if you've developed prediabetes.

Indeed, losing weight and boosting physical activity can delay or even prevent prediabetes from turning into T2DM and, in some cases, might normalize blood glucose levels. For example, in one study 'intensive lifestyle changes', such as losing at least 7 per cent of body weight and taking at least 150 minutes physical activity per week, reduced the risk that IGT would develop into diabetes by 58 per cent compared with the lifestyle advice doctors usually offered at the time of this study. Older people and those with a lower body mass index (BMI) showed a particular improvement, although everyone seemed to benefit.[10]

Body mass index

Weight isn't a very good guide to your risk of developing T2DM and other conditions linked to excess body fat. Weighing 14 stone (90 kg) is fine if you're 6 foot 5 inches (190 cm). But you would be seriously obese if you were 5 foot 6 inches (165 cm). So BMI is used to assess whether you're overweight or obese, based your height and weight. BMI estimates, roughly, your amount of body fat and, therefore, your risk of developing diseases linked to excess weight, such as heart disease, hypertension, T2DM, gall stones, breathing problems and some cancers. You should try to keep your BMI between 18.5 and 24.9 kg/m^2. Below this and you're dangerously underweight. A BMI between 25.0 and 29.9 kg/m^2 suggests that you are overweight. You're probably obese if your BMI exceeds 30.0 kg/m^2.

While BMI works for most people, it may overestimate body fat in athletes, body builders and other muscular people (such as those with manual jobs involving heavy lifting). On the other hand, BMI may underestimate body fat in older persons and people who have lost muscle. Your doctor can check your body fat level more accurately using a special monitor. The BMI of children and teenagers is slightly different. You can find a BMI chart for children and teens at <www.cdc.gov/healthyweight/assessing/bmi/childrens_bmi/about_childrens_bmi.html>.

It's worth making the effort. Diabetic complications (Chapter 4) can reduce life expectancy among people with T2DM by up to 10 years, according to Diabetes UK.

Other types of diabetes

Although T1DM and, particularly, T2DM together account for most cases of diabetes, there are also several less common types.

Gestational diabetes

Gestational diabetes occurs during approximately 1 in 20 pregnancies in the UK. Overweight and obese women are particularly likely to develop gestational diabetes, which usually emerges during the second or third trimester. In other women (especially cases that arise in the first trimester) the pregnancy uncovers pre-existing diabetes. Gestational diabetes usually arises because the pancreas doesn't produce enough insulin to meet the body's increased demands during pregnancy.

Gestational diabetes usually resolves after the baby's birth. However, around 30 per cent of women who develop gestational diabetes go on to develop T2DM – a rate three times higher than among the general population. Poorly controlled diabetes can also harm the unborn baby. So, it is especially important to ensure good control of blood glucose before and during pregnancy. It's also vital to make sure you take sufficient folic acid (folate) before and during the first trimester (page 108). Women planning a pregnancy and mums-to-be with diabetes need to take higher doses of this essential vitamin than healthy women.

Diabetes and the unborn child

Pregnant women with diabetes are five times more likely to have a stillbirth, Diabetes UK warns, than mothers-to-be with normal blood glucose levels. Their children are also three times more likely to die in the first few months of life. Furthermore, between 7 and 13 per cent of babies born to mothers with poorly controlled diabetes have a major congenital abnormality. This compares with between 2 and 3 per cent in those without diabetes. Good diabetes care can reduce the risk to about 1–5 per cent. Women with diabetes, especially if poorly controlled, are also more likely to give birth to an abnormally large baby.[3]

Maturity-onset diabetes of the young

Maturity-onset diabetes of the young (MODY) accounts for between 1 and 2 per cent of cases of diabetes. MODY tends to emerge before the age of 25 years and is a genetic disease that knocks out the beta cells' ability to sense changes in blood glucose levels.[3] MODY should not be confused with T2DM in young people.

A child born to a person with MODY has a 50 per cent chance of inheriting the affected gene and developing MODY. And 95 per cent of those that carry the MODY gene develop diabetes at some time.

Many people with MODY are probably misdiagnosed with T1DM or T2DM. Lifestyle changes, such as a healthier diet and increased physical activity, can treat many cases of MODY, so some people with T1DM may receive insulin injections they don't need. But check with your doctor before changing any medication.

Other causes of diabetes

Several diseases seem to increase the risk of developing diabetes. For example, calcium occasionally accumulates in the pancreas causing calcific diabetes.

Chronic (long-term) inflammation of the pancreas (pancreatitis) can destroy insulin-producing cells as well as being very painful and even life-threatening. Chronic pancreatitis causes between 0.5 and 1 per cent of cases of diabetes. Indeed, 40–60 per cent of those with chronic pancreatitis have diabetes. Pancreatitis can arise from high levels of fat (especially triglycerides – see page 8) in the blood and excessive alcohol consumption. But doctors can't find a cause for many cases of pancreatitis.[11]

Occasionally, drugs and surgery trigger diabetes. Secondary diabetes emerges immediately after surgeons remove a diseased pancreas, for example. Certain medicines can also trigger diabetes. Doctors realized many years ago that steroid tablets and thiazide diuretics ('water tablets' used to treat hypertension – dangerously raised blood pressure), although often lifesavers, potentially trigger diabetes. More recent studies suggest that inhaled steroids, especially at high doses, may also cause diabetes. One study included adults using inhaled corticosteroids (preventers) to treat asthma or chronic obstructive pulmonary disease (COPD). Over, on average, 5.5 years, inhaled corticosteroids increased the risk of developing diabetes by 34 per cent. Inhaled corticosteroids also increased the likelihood that people with diabetes would progress from antidiabetic tablets to insulin (suggesting that their diabetes got worse) by 34 per cent. The risk rose progressively with higher steroid doses.[12]

Diabetes insipidus, which affects about one in 25,000 people, arises when, for example, infection, injury or drugs, such as lithium used to treat bipolar disorder (manic depression), undermine the body's ability to regulate water levels. Affected people produce very large amounts of dilute, watery urine. And their urine doesn't taste sweet.

Symptoms

People with diabetes can develop a wide range of symptoms. Some of the hallmark symptoms of diabetes mellitus emerge as the body tries to deal with the high levels of glucose in the blood. For example, once glucose levels exceed about 12 mmol/l, the body tries to flush the excess out of the body. That's why people with diabetes mellitus urinate more (called polyuria) and their urine tastes sweet. Often, they tend to urinate more at night (nocturia) and, not surprisingly, tend to feel thirsty (polydipsia).

Other symptoms emerge because cells can't tap into this important source of energy. So people with diabetes (we'll assume from now on that diabetes means diabetes mellitus) can lose weight and feel weak. Indeed, without treatment, someone with T1DM can seem to be starving in the midst of plenty.

Unlike T2DM, the symptoms of T1DM tend to appear over several days to weeks. Nevertheless, the symptoms of T1DM develop more slowly in people aged over 30 years. This can lead to confusion and misdiagnosis, especially if the person is overweight. Indeed, around 1 in 10 adults diagnosed with T2DM shows markers of autoimmune T1DM.[5]

See your doctor if you have any of the symptoms below. There are also some less common symptoms. For example, several conditions, including high levels of insulin, can cause acanthosis nigricans – dark, thick velvety patches around the groin, neck, armpits and other body folds. This is caused by the initial rise in insulin levels in patients with T2DM and in those who are overweight. These high levels of insulin increase your skin cells' activity, leading to acanthosis nigricans.

Common symptoms of diabetes

- more frequent urination than usual, especially at night
- being very thirsty; drinking excessively
- feeling hungry (especially T1DM)
- extreme tiredness and constant fatigue
- unexplained and sudden weight loss
- genital itching or regular episodes of thrush
- cuts, sores and wounds that heal slowly
- skin infections (especially recurrent)
- blurred vision
- tingling and numbness in the hands and feet.

Finally, in many cases the first sign of diabetes is a potentially serious complication (Chapter 4). For example, the first sign of T1DM may be ketoacidosis – a potentially dangerous rise in blood sugar levels. In people with T2DM, a complication such as a heart attack or eye damage may be the first indication that they have developed the disease. So, it's important that you see your GP if you experience any of the symptoms of diabetes or are at particularly high risk – an issue we'll explore in the next chapter.

3

Risk factors for diabetes

We face risk factors for diabetes from the cradle to the grave. Some we can't do anything about – such as our genes. But many risk factors are within our control. For instance, a healthy, balanced diet reduces your risk of developing T2DM. There are too many risk factors to consider in detail, so in this chapter we'll look at the most important.

Obesity

A poor diet and lack of exercise are important modifiable causes of T2DM, in part because they increase the risk of being obese or overweight. Indeed, being overweight causes around 90 per cent of cases of T2DM. In the UK, around three-fifths of women and two-thirds of men are overweight or obese. Being overweight causes cosmetic problems. People may find the clothes they like don't suit their shape. Overweight people often feel lethargic and find exercise taxing, which helps the pounds pile on. But the problems posed by being overweight are more than skin deep. Excess weight is associated with numerous health issues, including:

- breathlessness;
- bowel problems;
- hypertension;
- raised levels of cholesterol and other harmful fats in the blood, which contribute to heart disease (page 44);
- some cancers, including colon, kidney and breast. According to the *British Journal of Cancer*, excess body weight was the third most common avoidable carcinogen (after smoking and diet), causing about 1 in every 18 cancers in the UK;[1]
- T2DM.

All these diseases in turn carry their own risk of serious complications.

The health burden imposed by excess weight is going to get even heavier. If current trends continue, another 11 million adults in the UK will be obese by 2030, resulting in 331,000 extra cases of coronary heart disease and stroke, 545,000 more cases of diabetes and 87,000 additional cancers. Being overweight is not a matter to take lightly.

Not all fat is equal

Broadly, the body produces two types of fat. A layer of subcutaneous fat just below the skin conserves body heat. Abdominal (visceral) fat is more biologically active than the subcutaneous layer. Indeed, far from being inert blubber, fat (which biologists call adipose tissue) is a biological factory continuously pumping out chemicals that carry messages around the body.

High levels of these chemicals are one reason why being overweight – even just carrying a few extra pounds – increases the risk of developing diabetes. As a result, the American Diabetes Association suggests that people who don't have symptoms of diabetes but who are overweight and over 45 years of age should be tested for diabetes or prediabetes.

On the other hand, if you can lose about 5–7 per cent of your weight – that's about 4.5–6.8 kg for someone who weighs 90 kg – you may be able to postpone T2DM. Try to lose weight slowly by changing your diet and increasing your activity level (see Chapter 6).

Ethnicity and waist size

T2DM usually occurs in obese and overweight people over 40 years of age. However, T2DM appears at an earlier age and is more common in certain ethnic groups. For example, in South Asian and black people, T2DM typically appears from the age of 25 years. Furthermore, Diabetes UK reports that T2DM is:

- up to six times more common in people of South Asian origin compared with white people and
- up to three times more common in people from African–Caribbean and African backgrounds compared with white people.

As a result, the cut-off for dangerous abdominal obesity is lower for people of some ethnic backgrounds, especially those of South Asian origin (Table 2).

Table 2 Waist sizes linked to increased risk of health problems

	Waist size	
	Heath at risk	Health at high risk
Men	Over 94 cm (37 inches)	Over 102 cm (40 inches)
Women	Over 80 cm (32 inches)	Over 88 cm (35 inches)
South Asian men	–	Over 90 cm (36 inches)
South Asian women	–	Over 80 cm (32 inches)

Source: Adapted from the British Heart Foundation

However, losing weight is tough. In the UK Prospective Diabetes Study (UKPDS) only 16 per cent of those recently diagnosed with diabetes reached their target fasting glucose level on diet alone after 3 months. Only half of these maintained their improved glucose levels for 1 year.[2] But try to lose as much weight as you can – every little helps.

Metabolic syndrome

You're more likely to develop T2DM if you're overweight than someone with a healthy BMI (page 18). In turn, you're more likely to develop dangerously raised blood pressure (hypertension) if you're overweight. And if you have diabetes, hypertension increases your risk of developing heart disease. In other words, risk factors cluster, creating a deadly combination. This cluster of risk factors, known as metabolic syndrome, is one reason why heart disease kills more people with diabetes than any other condition.

A deadly combination

The landmark INTERHEART study[3] compared 15,152 patients from 52 countries who had experienced their first heart attack with 14,820 people who had never had a heart attack. Researchers identified nine factors that accounted for 90 per cent of the risk of the first heart attack in men and 94 per cent among women (see Table 3). Eating fruits and vegetables daily (30 per cent reduction), regular exercise (14 per cent reduction) and regular alcohol consumption (9 per cent reduction) protected against the first heart attack. A healthy diet and exercise also helps control diabetes.

Table 3 Factors linked to the risk of suffering a first heart attack in the INTERHEART study

Risk factor	Increase in heart attack risk
Hypertension alone	1.9 times
Diabetes alone	2.4 times
Smoking alone	2.9 times
Abnormal lipid profile (dyslipidaemia)	3.3 times
Hypertension, diabetes, smoking	13.0 times
Hypertension, diabetes, smoking, dyslipidaemia	42.3 times
Hypertension, diabetes, smoking, dyslipidaemia, obesity	68.5 times
Hypertension, diabetes, smoking, dyslipidaemia, psychosocial factors	182.9 times
Hypertension, diabetes, smoking, dyslipidaemia, psychosocial factors, obesity	333.7 times

Source: Yusuf S, et al.[3]

INTERHEART also found that smoking just one to five cigarettes a day increased the risk of having a heart attack by 38 per cent compared with lifelong non-smokers. The risk roughly doubled in those smoking 6–10 cigarettes a day, increased almost fourfold between 16 and 20 a day, and rose to just over ninefold in people smoking at least 41 cigarettes a day. See page 72 for some tips on quitting smoking. Diabetes and hypertension each roughly doubled the risk of the first heart attack.

Importantly, INTERHEART showed how clusters of risk factors, including diabetes, dramatically increases the risk of heart attacks:

- People with diabetes who smoke and have hypertension are 13 times more likely to experience a heart attack than those without any of the nine risk factors.
- Those with diabetes and four other risk factors (harmful fat levels, obesity, smoking and hypertension) are almost 69 times more likely to have a heart attack.
- If you're unfortunate enough to endure psychosocial problems (such as stress and depression) in addition to diabetes and the other four risk factors you are about 334 times more likely to have a heart attack than those without any of the nine risk factors.

Defining the metabolic syndrome

Metabolic syndrome (previously called syndrome X and insulin resistance syndrome) can arise several years before the onset of diabetic symptoms or complications. So, people with metabolic syndrome are often prediabetic. Definitions vary, but if you have at least three of the following (continued overleaf), a doctor may diagnose metabolic syndrome:

- Diabetes or IFG (page 16), or you are taking a drug for diabetes (Chapter 5).
- A large waistline – abdominal obesity or an 'apple' shape – at least 94 cm in European men and at least 80 cm in European women. Cut-off points differ for certain ethnic groups (see Table 2 on page 25).
- Abnormal lipids (dyslipidaemia), such as low levels of high-density lipoprotein (HDL) in your blood, or you're taking a medicine (such as a fibrate or niacin – ask your GP or pharmacist if you're not sure) to boost levels of this 'healthy' fat.

Healthy and lethal cholesterol

Despite its bad press, cholesterol is an essential building block of the membranes that surround every cell. Cholesterol also forms part of the insulation around many nerve fibres (myelin sheath) that ensures signals travel properly. And cholesterol forms the backbone of several hormones, including oestrogen, testosterone and progesterone. But poor diets and a lack of exercise mean that many of us have too much of a good thing.

Transporting cholesterol around the body poses a problem: it is not soluble in water and blood is about four-fifths water. To be transported, cholesterol (and other oil-soluble substances such as fatty acids and triglycerides, collectively called lipids) must be bound to a protein that is soluble in water. These assemblies of proteins and lipids are called lipoproteins. One of these, LDL, carries cholesterol from the liver to the tissues. LDL accumulates in artery walls, forming fatty deposits called plaques that cause most heart attacks (page 44). Another, HDL, carries cholesterol away from the arteries and back to the liver for excretion, cutting heart attack risk. In other words, high LDL levels increase heart attack risk. High levels of HDL protect against heart attacks. It's easy to remember: LDL is 'lethal'; HDL is 'healthy'.

- High levels of triglycerides, or you're taking medicines to cut levels of this harmful fat.
- Hypertension, or you're taking a medicine to reduce your blood pressure.

Metabolic syndrome reminds us that risk factors for heart attacks commonly cluster. If you have one risk factor you should probably ask your GP or nurse to check for others – such as diabetes if you're carrying extra weight around your belly, or IFG if you have hypertension. Doctors and patients should treat each component of the metabolic syndrome appropriately and aggressively.

Alcohol and diabetes

Alcohol is a doubled-edged sword – for people with diabetes as well as society more widely. It's often part of celebrations, casual get-togethers and daily life. But although alcohol is legal, it's still a drug. Indeed, alcohol kills more people than street drugs. In England, 1,738 people died due to drug misuse in 2008. But there were 8,664 alcohol-related deaths in 2009, more than double the 4,023 recorded during 1992. The current death toll from alcohol is equivalent to a jumbo jet crashing every 17 days.

Alcohol is a relaxant, reduces inhibitions and, in moderation, ensures a good time in company. However, in larger amounts alcohol impairs reason, potentially (by reducing inhibitions) promotes aggression, and slows mental and physical reactions. And heavy drinking is linked to a range of serious diseases including liver disease, heart attacks, stroke and several malignancies. According to the *British Journal of Cancer*, alcohol causes around 1 in every 25 cancers.[1]

Unfortunately, the UK is a nation of heavy drinkers. But excessive drinking isn't just a problem for bingeing teenagers or homeless drunks. According to the Office for National Statistics, 41 per cent of men in managerial and professional households drank more than 4 units (see box) on at least 1 day in the previous week. And in these households, 35 per cent of women drank more than 3 units on at least 1 day in the week before interview. This compares with 34 per cent of men and 23 per cent of women in routine or manual-work households.

Alcohol can inflame the pancreas (page 20), causing pancrea-titis, as well as helping to pile on the pounds. So, not surprisingly, excessive alcohol consumption may increase the risk of devel-oping T2DM, especially among men. However, the relationship is complex. Indeed, moderate consumption may reduce T2DM risk by heightening cells' sensitivity to insulin, lowering circulating levels of insulin or both.[4]

For example, in a Swedish study, alcohol consumption and binge drinking increased the risk of prediabetes (by 42 per cent) and T2DM (by 67 per cent) in men. However, low consumption (1.5–4.7 g/day) decreased diabetes risk in women (by 59 per cent).[5] Another study found that men who drank more than 21 US 'drinks' a week (about 37 UK units) were 50 per cent more likely to develop dia-betes than those drinking one or fewer drinks per week. No such association emerged in women.[6]

A UK unit of alcohol

One UK unit of alcohol contains 8 g alcohol. So:

- Half a pint of normal strength beer, lager or cider equals 1 unit.
- One small (100 ml) glass of wine equals 1 unit.
- A large (175 ml) glass of wine equals 2 units.
- A single (25 ml) measure of spirits equals 1 unit.
- One 275 ml bottle of alcopop (5.5 percent/volume) equals 1.5 units.

A US 'drink' contains 14 g of alcohol.

Binge drinking in particular seems to increase diabetes risk. In one study, men who drank at least 210 g of alcohol over 1–3 days in the week before the study (that's about 13 pints of standard strength beer, cider or lager) were five times more likely to develop T2DM. But drinking this amount of alcohol over 4–7 days did not increase the risk of diabetes.[4] So if you have prediabetes or T2DM don't drink more than the recommended limits (page 88).

Alcohol poses other risks for people with diabetes. For example,

- If you're using insulin or antidiabetic tablets (especially a type called sulphonylureas – page 59) to control your blood glucose levels, you need to remain within the limits agreed with your diabetes team to avoid potentially dangerous hypoglycaemic attacks.

- Alcohol can increase levels of triglycerides. Many people with diabetes have high levels of these fats, which are linked to heart disease, in their blood.
- Alcohol can also exacerbate the pain from neuropathy caused by diabetes, and further damage the nerves.
- Regularly drinking more than 3–4 units of alcohol a day can exacerbate retinopathy.[7]

But that doesn't mean people with diabetes need to take the pledge. We'll look at how you can safely enjoy a drink in Chapter 6.

Polycystic ovary syndrome

Polycystic ovary syndrome (PCOS) usually occurs when certain hormones are in disarray. In women with PCOS numerous cysts, usually no bigger than 8 mm, develop around the edge of the ovaries. These cysts contain underdeveloped eggs. All women have some such cysts. But most women with PCOS have many more. In many cases, these follicles cannot release their egg.

The cause of PCOS remains rather enigmatic. All women produce small amounts of some supposedly 'male' hormones, such as testosterone. But those with PCOS either produce markedly higher levels or these male hormones are particularly active. Furthermore, many people with PCOS produce excessive levels of insulin, for example because they are overweight. The increased insulin levels seem to contribute to the increased production and activity of male hormones.

PCOS symptoms usually emerge in the late teens or early 20s when women experience menstrual problems, such as irregular or light periods, or none at all, or find that they can't conceive. Other women develop excessive body hair (hirsutism), weight gain, oily skin and acne, and hair loss. Later in life the obesity, hormone imbalances and insulin resistance characteristic of PCOS lead to an increased risk of hypertension, dyslipidaemia and diabetes. So if you have symptoms of PCOS or have been diagnosed with PCOS you should see your doctor and ask to be checked for diabetes.

Economic deprivation

People from economically deprived backgrounds seem more likely to develop diabetes than their more affluent counterparts. For example:

- At any particular age, people from the most deprived background are 2.5-fold more likely to develop diabetes than the average in the UK.
- Women from homes with the lowest incomes are at least four times more likely to develop diabetes than those from homes with the highest incomes.
- People from deprived backgrounds are more likely to develop complications once diabetes emerges.

Diabetes UK points out that several mutually reinforcing factors contribute to the link between poverty and diabetes and its complications, including:

- higher levels of obesity
- physical inactivity
- unhealthy diet
- smoking and poor control of blood pressure.

Although such deprivation needs action from government, a healthy diet and the other suggestions in this book could go a long way to reducing the risk of diabetes among some of the most vulnerable people in our society.

4

Complications of poorly controlled diabetes

The raised levels of blood glucose typical of diabetes can 'poison' cells, contributing to diabetic complications.[1] Most people with diabetes also show abnormalities in the way their body handles fat (dyslipidaemia), which contributes to strokes, heart attacks and gangrene in the feet.[2]

These complications take many years to emerge, offering you the opportunity to reduce your risk by sticking to any medications measuring your blood glucose level as recommended by your diabetes team, and following a healthy lifestyle. In general, complications start emerging between 7 and 10 years after the onset of T1DM.[3] Those linked to T2DM can take even longer to emerge. But as Robert Tattersall remarks, while doctors once described T2DM as mild diabetes, because patients did not usually need insulin, the complications in type 2 diabetes can be as serious or even worse than in type 1.[2]

Microvascular and macrovascular complications

Doctors broadly separate diabetic complications into microvascular and macrovascular:

- Microvascular complications include neuropathy (nerve damage), nephropathy (kidney disease) and retinopathy (damage to the light-sensitive layer at the back of eye).
- Macrovascular complications include heart disease, stroke and peripheral vascular disease – a blockage in the blood vessels supplying the limbs, which can end in gangrene and even amputation of the toes, feet and lower leg.
- Other complications of diabetes include a higher risk of infections, impotence, problems during pregnancy and, in children, impaired growth and development.

The benefits of tight control

Tightly controlling blood glucose reduces the risk of complications in T1DM and T2DM. For example, the Diabetes Control and Complications Trial (DCCT) compared intensive and standard treatment (at the time of the study) in people with T1DM. Patients in the intensive therapy group measured their blood glucose levels four times a day. Based on these measurements, they adjusted their insulin dose to, for example, keep blood glucose levels before meals to 3.9–6.7 mmol/l and HbA_{1c} (a longer term measure of blood glucose control; page 37) to less than 6.05 per cent (43 mmol/mol). People with T1DM following standard treatment aimed to avoid hyperglycaemia, ketones in their urine and severe or frequent hypoglycaemia. They did not generally change their insulin dose each day.

Intensive therapy reduced the risk of developing:

- retinopathy by 76 per cent;
- kidney damage by 39–54 per cent;
- nerve damage by 60 per cent.

However, severe hypoglycaemia was between two and three times more common in the intensive arm.[4] The take-home message is that tight control reduces damage to your eyes, kidneys and nerves.

Researchers published the results of DCCT in 1993 and standard treatment has improved dramatically since then – driven by these compelling results and those from other studies. Modern standard treatment is much closer to the intensive therapy in DCCT.

And it's a similar story in T2DM. A study called UKPDS 35 found that in people with T2DM, each 1 per cent decline in HbA_{1c} reduced:

- the risk of heart attacks by 14 per cent;
- deaths related to diabetes by 21 per cent;
- microvascular complications by 37 per cent.[5]

The need to tightly control your blood glucose levels and avoid complications linked to, for example, eating excessive amounts of fat is one reason why a healthy, balanced diet is essential for everyone with diabetes.

Checking blood glucose levels

Raised blood glucose levels only rarely cause symptoms – a potentially serious condition called hyperglycaemia. So, your diabetes team may suggest that you check your levels regularly using a self-testing kit. This is essential if you're using insulin or some other treatments for T2DM. Your team may also suggest that you monitor your blood glucose levels in some other circumstances, such as helping to determine when a person with T2DM needs to start antidiabetic tablets or move from tablets to insulin.

Measuring blood glucose can seem daunting at first. However, in time, testing becomes second nature and helps:

- Ensure you're taking the right dose of insulin for your diet, exercise levels and so on.
- Detect dangerously high glucose levels (hyperglycaemia).
- Detect dangerously low glucose levels (hypoglycaemia), which can pose a problem with insulin and some oral glucose-lowering medications (Chapter 5).
- Assess the impact of changes to your diet.
- Determine whether an illness, such as an infection, undermines control of your blood glucose levels.
- Help plan and assess any impact of changes in exercise and physical activity.
- Examine changes in blood glucose over time – such as whether your diabetes is getting worse or lifestyle changes are improving control.
- Decide whether you need to change your medication and assess whether the new drug regimen improves control.
- To ensure safety while driving or during other activities.

However, blood glucose levels change constantly over the course of the day as we digest food and our activity levels change. The blood glucose measurement can only tell you the level at that time. That's why your diabetes team takes another reading (called HbA_{1c} – see page 37) that takes an average of your blood glucose level over 3 months.

Over time, you'll see how changes in your lifestyle, such as a healthy balanced diet, influence your blood glucose levels. Keeping a diary of your blood glucose readings will help. As Diabetes UK notes, some blood glucose monitoring devices store readings. But keeping a diary also allows you to note your activities at the time you took the measurement, what you ate and how you felt. You'll gradually gain the confidence to make changes that allow you to control your diabetes rather than letting your diabetes control you.

Making blood glucose measurements easier

A blood glucose monitor uses a very sharp needle, called a lancet, to release a drop of blood. A sophisticated monitor then measures the amount of glucose. Not surprisingly, many people find even the thought of being stabbed with a lancet unpleasant. Actually, most people get used to the jab; the thought is usually worse than the experience. But you can make life a little easier. Diabetes UK suggests washing your hands in warm water first or giving your hands a good shake; both increase blood flow to your hands. And choose the least painful site. Lancing the side of the finger is often less painful than jabbing the sensitive fingertip, for example. Some devices allow you to take a sample from the upper arm or thigh, which are less sensitive than the finger – ask your doctor or diabetes nurse for more details. Finally, some people find certain devices less painful than others. Again, your doctor or diabetes nurse can help you find the blood test device that's right for you.

Measuring and adapting your treatment to tightly control your blood glucose level helps reduce the risk of complications. Nevertheless, you should still see your doctor at least once a year to check:

- your feet and legs to see if your feet are becoming numb, which is a sign of neuropathy (page 49);
- your blood pressure: hypertension increases the risk of heart attacks, strokes and kidney disease;
- your cholesterol (LDL, HDL [see page 27] and total) and tri-glyceride concentrations: as mentioned above, dyslipidaemia is a leading cause of cardiovascular disease among people with diabetes;
- your kidneys: persistently high blood glucose levels can damage your kidneys (page 47) leading to protein 'leaking' into your urine. Doctors call this condition, depending on the level of protein, microalbuminuria or albuminuria.

You should also see your optician – at least once a year but more often if you have diabetic eye disease – and dentist regularly. Make sure they know you have diabetes.

Urine testing

Testing your urine is less painful than using a lancet to draw blood. Unfortunately, measuring glucose in urine is less accurate than testing blood. So, urine testing may miss subtle but potentially important changes in blood glucose levels. Indeed, the body tries to flush excess glucose out of the body once blood levels exceed about 12 mmol/l. But this is far higher than the levels that can cause complications. As Diabetes UK points out, your urine test should always be negative. Even a trace of glucose in your urine means that your blood levels are too high. Furthermore, some people with normal blood glucose levels excrete sugar in their urine, either during pregnancy or because they have a relatively rare genetic condition called renal glycosuria.[2] In other words, whenever possible, it's best to measure blood glucose levels.

Your blood glucose target

Your diabetes team will help you decide the right testing regimen for you. If you have T1DM, you'll probably need to test your blood glucose levels several times a day. Your doctor or diabetes nurse will agree an individual target for your blood glucose level. Table 4 shows some typical targets, but as everyone is different you may find these vary from those agreed with your doctor or diabetes nurse.

Table 4 Typical blood glucose targets

	Before meals	Two hours after eating
T1DM in adults	4–7 mmol/l	No more than 9 mmol/l
T2DM in adults	4–7 mmol/l	No more than 8.5 mmol/l
Pregnancy	3.5–5.9 mmol/l	No more than 7.8 mmol/l 1 hour after eating
Children (under 16 years) T1DM	4–8 mmol/l	No more than 10 mmol/l
Children (under 16 years) T2DM	Your doctor or diabetes nurse will set an individual target	

Source: Adapted from Diabetes UK

Once your diabetes team sets your target, you'll need to discover for yourself how the foods you eat and your levels of activity influence your blood glucose levels. Everyone's different. Regular testing and keeping a food diary (page 74) should give you a clearer picture of your body's response to different foods. If you find that certain foods raise your blood glucose, try to eat them less often, dish up a smaller portion size or even eliminate this food (assuming of course it's not an essential source of nutrients – your dietician can help).

Likewise, the effect of exercise on blood glucose levels varies from person to person. When you exercise, your cells need more fuel. So, your cells use more glucose and their insulin resistance declines. This means you should test your blood glucose level when you work out and adjust your insulin dose or eat more carbohydrate to keep within your target range.[6] It's especially important to monitor your levels carefully when you start a new workout or even when your day-to-day exercise increases, such as moving from sitting in front of computer screen in an office to a more active holiday.

To err is human and everyone with diabetes slips up from time to time. It's easy to forget to record your readings if you're busy juggling diabetes, family life and a career. It's easy to eat too much, especially if you are distracted by family and friends – or just cannot resist the temptation. And your body may not play ball, sometimes burning off too much, or not enough, glucose for no apparent reason. But don't be tempted to fabricate the results of your blood glucose levels, even if you're worried about criticism from your doctor or nurse. Paternalistic 'Sir Lancelot Spratts' are anachronisms. Modern healthcare professionals know how difficult living with diabetes can be, they are sympathetic and can help you, but only if they know your real blood glucose levels and how well you stick to the lifestyle suggestions and medicines.

HbA$_{1c}$: A different perspective

As mentioned above, a blood glucose measurement tells you the level at that time. It doesn't take account of the peaks and troughs over the course of the days, weeks and months. As a result, your doctor or diabetes nurse will measure your HbA$_{1c}$ (glycosylated haemoglobin) level at least once a year. HbA$_{1c}$ measures the amount of glucose carried by red blood cells. Glucose 'sticks' to the haemoglobin that carries oxygen; the technical term is glycosylation. Red blood cells don't rely on transporters (page 7) to move glucose into the cell. So, measuring HbA_{1c} indicates your blood glucose levels for the previous 2–3 months – the lifespan of the haemoglobin molecule.

A new way of reporting HbA_{1c}

Until recently, doctors reported HbA_{1c} levels as a percentage. However, they are now switching to a measure called millimoles per mol (mmol/mol). An HbA_{1c} of 6.5 per cent translates into 48 mmol/mol (see Table 5). Diabetes UK offers a calculator to convert HbA_{1c} levels as a percentage into mmol/mol at: <www.diabetes.org. uk/hba1c>.

To reduce the risk of diabetic complications, you should aim to keep HbA_{1c} below 6.5 per cent (48 mmol/mol). But if you're at risk of severe hypoglycaemia your diabetes team may suggest a target of less than 7.5 per cent (58 mmol/mol). However, HbA_{1c} measurements aren't an infallible guide to diabetes-related risk. For example:

- Certain diseases of the blood, including anaemia, thalassaemia and sickle cell disease, can give anomalous readings.[7]
- The risk of eye damage (retinopathy) increases once HbA_{1c} exceeds 6.0 per cent (42 mmol/mol) to 6.4 per cent (46 mmol/ mol).
- HbA_{1c} doesn't distinguish T1DM from T2DM, reflect day-to-day changes in blood glucose control or the impact of diet or exercise.[3]

In other words, you need both HbA_{1c} and regular blood glucose measurements to provide the most accurate picture of your diabetes control and the impact of changes to your drugs, lifestyle and diet.

Hypoglycaemia

Hypoglycaemia (sometimes spelt hypoglycemia) occurs when blood sugar falls to dangerously low levels – 'hypo' means 'under'. At blood glucose levels under about 4 mmol/l, there isn't enough glucose to fuel your body's activities, which can cause a range of symptoms (see box opposite). However, each person shows a

Table 5 Equivalent values of HbA$_{1c}$

Mmol/mol	Per cent
42	6.0
48	6.5
53	7.0
59	7.5
64	8.0
69	8.5
75	9.0
80	9.5
86	10.0
91	10.5
97	11.0
102	11.5
108	12.0

Some common symptoms of hypoglycaemia

Early symptoms:
- hunger
- sweating
- shaking and trembling
- weakness
- rapid heartbeat, fast pulse, palpitations
- numb and tingling in and around the lips
- headache
- blurred vision
- dizziness
- looking pale.

Intermediate symptoms:
- difficulties with thinking and concentrating
- double vision
- poor coordination
- fatigue
- confusion
- irritability, nervousness, anxiety.

Late symptoms:
- unconsciousness
- seizures.

Adapted and expanded from Mazze[3]

unique pattern of hypo-related symptoms and these can change over time in the same person.

Almost all cases of hypoglycaemia arise from poor coordination between the dose of insulin and eating or activity.[6] Some antidiabetic tablets are also especially prone to trigger hypos; see Chapter 5. So Diabetes UK warns that you may be especially likely to develop hypos if you:

- delay or miss a meal or snack;
- don't eat enough carbohydrate;
- take part in unplanned or especially strenuous activity;
- drink too much alcohol, especially on an empty stomach.

The lack of food overnight can trigger hypos. Blood glucose varies in everyone during the day, usually reaching the lowest level between 2 a.m. and 3 a.m. Not surprisingly, hypos are most likely around this time. Changing the type of insulin you use (see Chapter 5) can help prevent nocturnal hypos.[6]

Often there's no obvious trigger for the hypo. However, keeping a diary of your blood glucose readings, when hypos occur and the associated symptoms can help you indentify whether you and your diabetes team can improve your control.

Treating hypoglycaemia

If untreated, severe hypoglycaemia can end in unconsciousness, coma or a fit. So, if you have any of the symptoms in the box (page 39) or your blood glucose measurements suggest you're at risk of a hypo (in most people less than 4 mmol/l), you should immediately consume between 10 and 20 g of a rapidly acting carbohydrate, such as:

- a glass of Lucozade, a non-diet soft drink or fruit juice;
- at least three glucose tablets (it's a good idea to carry these with you);
- five jelly babies or other sweets;
- two tablespoons (20 g) of dried fruit, honey or syrup.

The exact amount of carbohydrate needed to restore normal blood glucose levels varies from person to person and over time in the same person. So, you should test your blood glucose levels again after 15 minutes. If your blood glucose is still too low, consume another 10–20 g of rapidly acting carbohydrate.

Once you're back in the target range you should eat some long-acting carbohydrates to stop your blood glucose from falling again. Again, the exact amount varies from person to person. But if your next meal isn't due in the 15 minutes after you're back in the target range, Diabetes UK suggests eating one of the following:

- half a sandwich
- some fruit
- a small bowl of cereal – carry some cereal bars or fruit with you
- biscuits and milk.

Hyperglycaemia and ketoacidosis

As we saw in Chapter 1, the body keeps blood glucose levels within a relatively narrow range. Symptoms of hyperglycaemia can arise if blood levels rise too high.

Typical symptoms of hyperglycaemia

- increased thirst
- frequent urination
- lethargy/lack of energy
- headaches
- stomach pain.

Source: Diabetes UK

Again, numerous factors can trigger hyperglycaemia, Diabetes UK comments, including:

- missing a dose of insulin;
- using insufficient insulin;
- eating more carbohydrate than usual;
- over-treating hypoglycaemia;
- stress;
- infections.

So, you need to flush the excess glucose from your body by drinking large amounts of sugar-free fluids and you may need another dose of insulin. You'll also need to test for ketoacidosis (see page 42). If you experience attacks regularly, you may need to look at your diet, such as cutting back on cakes and sugary drinks. Regular exercise also helps maintain healthy blood sugar levels.

Ketoacidosis

As we saw in Chapter 1, when cells can't use glucose as a source of energy the body begins to 'burn' fat. However, switching to fat creates a group of by-products called ketones (sometimes called ketone bodies), which include acetoacetate, acetone and beta-hydroxybutyrate. Ketones can act as a source of fuel. Even the brain can use ketones when there is no glucose available.

However, ketones are toxic. So, the body immediately starts excreting them in urine. That's why people who produce large amounts of ketones often become increasingly thirsty. But if you produce more ketones than your body can handle, you may develop a potentially serious condition called ketoacidosis. Ketones are acids, so as they accumulate the blood becomes increasingly acidic. You may start feeling nauseous or vomit, your skin feels dry, your eyesight blurs and you take deep, rapid breaths. However, vomiting dehydrates the body, which hinders the kidney's ability to flush out ketones. In response, ketone levels rise even more rapidly.

Symptoms of ketoacidosis

- frequent urination
- excessive thirst
- increased appetite
- abdominal pain or discomfort
- heavy, deep (called Kussmaul) breathing
- vomiting
- dehydration
- acetone on the breath
- confusion and lethargy.

Adapted from Mazze[3]

As ketone levels rise, the breath may smell similar to pear drops or nail polish (nail polish contains acetone, which smells similar to pear drops). Finally, the combination of raised ketones and high blood glucose levels produces a potentially fatal coma. So, rapid treatment is essential.

People using insulin are especially prone to developing diabetic ketoacidosis. If you have T1DM your diabetes care team will advise when you need to check your ketone levels, usually by dipping a testing strip into a fresh urine sample. You may, however, be offered an electronic device that can detect ketones in blood. These devices show rising ketone levels 2–4 hours sooner than measurements using urine.[3] In rare cases, people controlling their diabetes with diet or tablets develop ketoacidosis. The risk is particularly high when they fall ill.

Diabetes UK suggests that people with diabetes should test their urine for ketones when their blood glucose level exceeds 15 mmol/l or if they have any symptoms of ketoacidosis. If the test strips indicate that your ketone levels are high (especially if your blood glucose levels are also raised) you should call your doctor or diabetes nurse immediately or go to your nearest casualty department. If your ketone levels are high and you feel very unwell – if you feel drowsy, breathless or nauseous, or you are vomiting – go directly to A&E. Ask another person to take you or ring for an ambulance.

Diabetes and infections

People with diabetes are especially vulnerable to infections for two main reasons. First, high blood sugar levels can undermine the immune system. Second, bacteria and fungi – such as the yeast that causes thrush – use sugars to fuel their growth.[7]

White blood cells and other cells in your body use a lot of energy when they tackle illness and fight infections. So, during illness and infections your body releases more glucose into the blood and some cells respond less well to insulin. These changes occur even if you lose your appetite or are off your food entirely. In other words, you should not stop taking your insulin and Diabetes UK recommends that you test your blood glucose level at least four times a day while you feel under the weather. You should ask your GP or diabetes nurse for more advice if you're worried. It's also worth making sure that a close family member or friend knows how to check your blood glucose levels and adjust your medication in case you feel too sick to take the measurement. You should always wear a medical alert bracelet to inform people of your condition – if you're unconscious, for example. If you don't have one, ask your GP or diabetes nurse.

Diabetes and heart disease

T2DM shortens life expectancy by up to 10 years, largely because of a dramatically increased risk of developing diseases affecting the heart and blood vessels. Such cardiovascular disease kills 44 per cent of people with T1DM and 52 per cent of those with T2DM, Diabetes UK warns. People with diabetes are also roughly twice as likely to have a stroke in the 5 years after their doctor has diagnosed diabetes. Atherosclerosis – where fatty deposits fur up your arteries – is responsible for most of the increased risk.

Overall, diabetes increases your risk of coronary heart disease (which includes angina and heart attacks, but not stroke or heart failure) between two- and fourfold. One study examined people who had not previously experienced a heart attack. Approximately 4 per cent of those without diabetes had their first heart attack over the next 7 years. But the rate was about five times higher in those with T2DM (19 per cent). T2DM also more than doubled the risk of a further heart attack in those who survived a heart attack (20 and 45 per cent in those without and with diabetes, respectively).[8]

Diabetes also dramatically cuts your chance of surviving a heart attack. After allowing for other risk factors, such as age, sex, smoking and treatments, death rates following heart attacks are a third higher among people with diabetes.[9]

The development of plaques

Even in people without diabetes, fatty material starts collecting inside our arteries from early childhood, and sometimes while we are still in the womb. Over the years, these deposits develop into the atherosclerotic plaques that are the main cause of heart attacks. 'Sclerosis' means hardening and 'athere' is Greek for gruel or porridge, which gives you an idea of the consistency – a hard cap covers the fatty core. As a plaque enlarges, the lumen of the blood vessel (the bore down the middle of the vessel) narrows. The reduced blood supply can cause a range of health problems depending on the site of the plaque, including chest pain (angina), kidney damage and impotence.

Plaques form around damage to the blood vessel's normally smooth inner lining. Numerous risk factors can damage the delicate lining and sow the seeds of atherosclerosis, including:

- diabetes
- excessive levels of fat in the blood
- dangerously high blood pressure
- changes linked to age
- nicotine and other toxins from smoking.

The damage triggers a sequence of events that leads to the development of an atherosclerotic plaque (Figure 3).

The damage to the vessel's inner lining allows fats and certain types of white blood cell to enter the vessel wall. Some of the white blood cells engorge with fat, forming foam cells. Meanwhile, chemicals released by white blood cells promote inflammation around the damaged area and increase the amount of muscle and collagen (which enhances strength and flexibility) in the blood vessel wall. The chemicals also recruit even more white blood cells into the damaged area.

These changes help patch the damaged vessel wall. But it's a short-term fix. As fat continues to pour from the blood into the plaque, muscle cells form a cap covering a core of foam cells, lipid and debris from dead cells. Capillaries grow into the developing plaque. But these vessels are fragile, so blood leaks into, and further swells, the plaque. Calcium deposits gradually harden the plaque.

Some atherosclerotic plaques can burst or crack, spilling their contents into the vessel and triggering a blood clot. If the clot

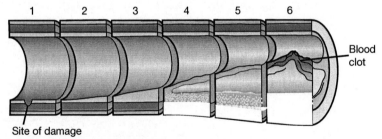

1 Damage to the inner lining of the blood vessel
2 Fatty streak forms at site of damage
3 Foam cells numbers increase, inflammation and small pools of fat appear
4 Large core of fat develops, and amounts of muscle and collagen increase
5 Fibrous cap covers a fat-rich core, while calcium deposits harden the plaque
6 Plaque ruptures triggering a blood clot

Figure 3 Development of an atherosclerotic plaque

forms in the vessel supplying the heart you'll probably suffer a heart attack. If the clot forms in the vessels supplying your brain you could have a stroke.

Peripheral arterial disease

If the plaque develops in a vessel supplying your legs – a condition called peripheral arterial (or vascular) disease – you may develop intermittent claudication (from the Latin for 'to limp').

Patients with intermittent claudication report aching or cramping pain, with tightness or fatigue in their leg muscles or buttocks. Some people find pain arises only during strenuous activity. People with more severe peripheral arterial disease may develop intermittent claudication after walking only a few metres. The pain subsides after a few minutes' rest.

Severe blockages to the blood flow to the legs can cause gangrene (tissue death), which may even end in amputation (page 50). One person in every three with atherosclerotic plaques in the heart's blood supply has peripheral arterial disease affecting their legs. Indeed, intermittent claudication can emerge before chest symptoms, warning you that you're especially likely to suffer a heart attack. So, tell your doctor if you have leg pain when you walk or climb stairs.

A balanced diet, especially as part of a healthy lifestyle, will dramatically reduce your risk of heart attack, stroke and peripheral vascular disease. Furthermore, your doctor may prescribe one or more drugs to reduce your risk, such as tablets to lower blood pressure (which can trigger plaque rupture) or reduce levels of dangerous fats in your blood. There's not space to look at the various options here, although you could try *The Heart Attack Survival Guide* by Mark Greener or look at the British Heart Foundation website (see Useful addresses) for more information.

Chronic kidney disease

Your kidneys filter your blood, keeping useful salts and water, and expelling waste products. As they control the amount of fluid and some salts, the kidneys help control blood pressure. However, in the UK, diabetes and hypertension are the leading causes of chronic kidney disease (nephropathy), which affects about 1 in 13 of the population.

As mentioned, the kidneys of people with diabetes attempt to normalize blood glucose levels by excreting sugar in urine. However, high levels of glucose in the blood can damage the tiny vessels inside the kidneys that filter the blood. Hypertension also damages these tiny vessels. As a result, the kidneys don't work effectively, which can eventually lead to nephropathy. Because diabetes and hypertension undermine the kidneys' ability to excrete waste and superfluous fluid, the extra fluid stays in the circulation, which pushes blood pressure even higher. Unless hypertension or diabetes is treated, the cycle of damage may leave the person needing a kidney transplant or dialysis. On the other hand, controlling blood pressure and glucose levels reduces the risk of kidney damage.

Testing for kidney damage

Most of us are born with more kidney function than we need. That's why living donors have healthy and full lives despite giving one of their kidneys to someone else. This reserve capacity also means that mild chronic kidney disease doesn't cause symptoms and often remains undiagnosed. As a result, up to 1 in 10 of us could have kidney disease. However, as the damage progresses you may develop one or more of the symptoms below. So, see your doctor if you develop any of these symptoms:

- tiredness
- swollen ankles, feet or hands caused by water retention
- shortness of breath
- itchy skin
- nausea
- problems having or keeping an erection.

Doctors and nurses can test for kidney disease with a simple urine test that detects protein. If you have kidney disease you begin to excrete protein in your urine – a condition called albuminuria or proteinuria. Small increases in levels of albumin (the most common protein in blood) in the urine (microalbuminuria) can identify early kidney disease long before you develop symptoms. Certain drugs – including angiotensin-converting enzyme (ACE) inhibitors and angiotensin receptor antagonists – seem to slow the progression of kidney disease. So, it's worth checking whether you've been tested recently.

Impotence and erectile dysfunction

Impotence is common among men with diabetes. Estimates vary, partly depending on the group of men studied and the method used, but between 35 and 90 per cent of men with diabetes experience erectile dysfunction – a failure to gain or keep an erection hard enough for sexual intercourse. In a large study from the USA, erectile dysfunction (sometimes called impotence) was three times more common in diabetic than non-diabetic men. Furthermore, while the risk of developing erectile dysfunction rises as all men get older, impotence typically emerges 10–15 years earlier in diabetic men.[10]

Several conditions linked to diabetes seem to increase the risk of erectile dysfunction, including raised levels of cholesterol and other fats, hypertension and obesity. Moreover, men with other diabetic complications, such as neuropathy, nephropathy, retinopathy and peripheral vascular disease, are also especially prone to develop erectile dysfunction. Finally, several medications (including some drugs used to treat hypertension), smoking and excessive alcohol intake can worsen diabetic erectile dysfunction.[10] Doctors can now offer Viagra (sildenafil) and a growing range of other treatments for erectile dysfunction. So swallow any embarrassment and speak to your doctor.

Sexual problems and diabetes in women

Up to a quarter of women with diabetes experience sexual dysfunction, including pain during intercourse and changes in desire, arousal or orgasm. Urinary tract infections and vaginal thrush – which are more common among women with diabetes – can contribute to these difficulties. Female sexual problems linked to diabetes are less well studied than those affecting men. However, these problems may be around twice as common in women with diabetes than in women generally. Doctors, nurses and counsellors can often resolve the problems.[7] So again, try to overcome your embarrassment.

ITEMS ISSUED/RENEWED
FOR Ms Asha Patel
ON 26/09/12 13:59:19
AT Idea Store Canary Wharf (IH)

Diabetes Healing Diet/Crabbes-Hinton, Chr
91000080250548 DUE 17/10/17

Prague/
91000080090551 DUE 17/10/17

Vienna/le Nevez, Catherine
91000080250492 DUE 17/10/17

3 Item(s) Issued

Nerve damage

Up to half of people with diabetes develop nerve damage (neuropathy), according to Diabetes UK. This damage can hinder the transmission of nerve signals from the brain and spinal cord to muscles, skin, the cardiovascular system and other organs, and vice versa, potentially causing severe pain and, as we'll see, leaving you vulnerable to potentially debilitating complications. The nerve damage can also cause 'autonomic' symptoms, which include constipation, diarrhoea, impotence, dry skin and poor awareness of hypoglycaemia. On the other hand, intensive blood glucose control more than halves the risk of neuropathy (57 per cent reduction) compared with less rigorous treatment (in other words, conventional treatment at the time of the study).[11]

Painful diabetic neuropathy

Neuropathy can cause considerable pain. Indeed, people with diabetes are around three times more likely to develop chronic painful neuropathy than the general population – 16 per cent and 5 per cent respectively.[12] Good control of blood sugar may prevent, partially reverse and slow progression of painful diabetic neuropathy.[13] Doctors can suggest a range of painkillers (analgesics) and other treatments for painful neuropathy. So if you feel discomfort see your GP.

Foot ulcers and amputations

Diabetes can damage the nerves that carry messages from your feet to your brain. This means that you may not realize when you tread on something sharp, develop a blister due to tight footwear or that the bath is too hot. As a result, you're more likely to suffer minor cuts, bruises or blisters and you're less likely to protect these small wounds by not walking on them. Indeed, you may not realize that a stone in your shoe is burrowing into the sole of your foot. This damage can quickly worsen and develop into ulcers – especially as the skin may not heal as well in people with diabetes.

Foot ulcers are common among people with diabetes. Between 15 and 25 per cent of people with diabetes develop at least one foot ulcer at some time. Between 1 and 4 per cent develop a foot ulcer in any year. So, at any time 4–10 per cent of people with diabetes have foot ulcers.[11]

Severe foot ulcers can lead to limb amputations, which are 10–30 times more common in people with diabetes than among the general population.[11] As mentioned above, a blocked artery supplying a limb can also lead to the cells dying, causing gangrene, especially in the toes. Again, this can lead to amputation. Diabetes UK warns that up to 70 per cent of people die within 5 years of undergoing an amputation because of their diabetes.

A growing problem

The growing number of people with diabetes is fuelling a marked rise in the number of amputations. For example, between 1996 and 2005, the number of 'minor' amputations (such as a toe) due to T1DM and those unrelated to diabetes declined by 11 per cent and 32 per cent, respectively. 'Major' amputations (such as the lower leg below the knee) declined by 41 per cent and 22 per cent, respectively, over this time. By contrast, the number of minor amputations related to T2DM performed in England almost doubled, while the number of major amputations increased by 43 per cent.[14]

However, myths and misconceptions surround this common problem. For example, many people with T2DM regard poor blood circulation, rather than foot ulcers, as the main cause of lower limb numbness, discomfort and amputation. So, they often try to improve the blood supply to their feet. One study found that half of people with diabetes regularly walked barefoot. Others wore open-toed sandals (with socks in the winter) or footwear a size too large 'to give the toes space to move'. Ironically, walking barefoot, or wearing sandals or poorly fitting shoes, could increase the chance that they will injure their feet.[15]

The risk of foot ulcers underscores why you need to see a chiropodist, podiatrist or foot protection team regularly. If you don't have any risk factors, for example, if the nerves in your feet still seem to transmit sensations normally, you may only need a once-yearly assessment. People with neuropathy and who have previously developed an ulcer, or have skin changes that could herald ulcers (such as dry skin, or red or yellowish discolouration) may need an assessment every 1–3 months.

Your GP, nurse or health visitor may be able to refer you to an NHS or private clinic and, if necessary, arrange a home visit. If you decide to find a chiropodist make sure that they are:

- specifically trained in diabetes;
- registered with the Health Professions Council;
- belong to the British Chiropody and Podiatry Association, the Society of Chiropodists and Podiatrists, or the Institute of Chiropodists and Podiatrists (see Useful addresses).

Between appointments, inspect your feet each day for cuts and splits between your toes or discolouration to your feet and toes – and see your doctor as soon as possible if these problems emerge.

Eye disease

Diabetes is the main cause of blindness among people of working age in the UK. Patients with diabetes are between 10 and 20 times more likely to go blind than people with normal blood glucose levels. Around 1 in every 50 people with diabetes will develop serious problems with their vision.[7]

Tragically, poorly controlled diabetes can damage the nerves in the hands. So, people left blind from diabetes may not be able to read Braille.[2] However, according to the Royal National Institute of Blind People (RNIB), early detection and treatment would prevent 90 per cent of cases of blindness caused by diabetes.

Diabetes increases the risk of several eye diseases. For example, people with diabetes are twice as likely as the rest of the population to develop cataracts (cloudiness in the lens) or glaucoma (increased pressure exerted by the fluid inside the eye, which eventually damages the retina). Furthermore, 20 years after their diagnosis, nearly everyone with T1DM and 60 per cent of those with T2DM have some degree of retinopathy, Diabetes UK says. Thirty per cent of people with T2DM show retinopathy by the time they are diagnosed.[16]

Retinopathy occurs when high blood levels of glucose damage the tiny blood vessels (capillaries) supplying the retina, the light-sensitive layer at the back of the eye. As a result, blood, fluid and fat leak into the retina. New blood vessels form as the body tries to bypass the damage. But these immature vessels are fragile and may burst. Blood flows into the eye causing sudden loss of vision. Over time, scar tissue can push the retina from the underlying tissue.[16]

Opticians and doctors can see early signs of retinopathy – soft accumulations of fluid called cotton-wool spots and changes to the shape of the capillaries – by examining your eyes.[16] These changes occur even before your vision alters, which is why it's so important that people with diabetes have their eyes checked each year.

Depression and anxiety

As long ago as the 1920s, doctors recognized that mental, social and familial problems contributed to marked fluctuations in blood glucose levels in certain people with diabetes. Indeed, some patients deliberately or subconsciously triggered hypoglycaemia or ketoacidosis as a way to avoid difficult situations at home by 'escaping' into hospital. More recently, people with eating disorders under-dosed on insulin to allow them to eat without gaining weight.[2] Meanwhile, doctors have increasingly recognized the sometimes heavy psychological burden imposed by living with a chronic disease such as diabetes.

Diabetic complications can be distressing and debilitating. If you experience a potentially fatal complication, such as a heart attack or stroke, you may live in fear for your life. Diabetes, especially if severe or poorly controlled, can cause considerable anxiety. And the need to tightly control blood glucose can impose a considerable mental toll, especially as people need to juggle their other commitments or feel guilty about the time they spend managing their disease or the impact on their families.

Given this, it's perhaps not surprising that depression is about twice as common in people with diabetes than in the rest of the population. In one study, individuals using insulin were 47 per cent more likely to receive antidepressants than people of the same age and sex without diabetes. The likelihood of requiring antidepressants was highest (around a fourfold increase) in people aged 30–39 years taking antidiabetic tablets or insulin.[17] People with diabetes are also more likely to develop anxiety, eating disorders and phobias.

Don't underestimate depression or anxiety

Depression is more than feeling 'down in the dumps'. It's profound, debilitating mental and physical lethargy, a pervasive sense of worthlessness and intense, deep, unshakeable sadness. Likewise, anxiety is more than feeling a little wound up, worried or stressed out. It's intense, sometimes debilitating, fear – even abject terror. If you've never experienced 'clinical' depression or anxiety, it's difficult to appreciate how devastating the conditions are.

In some cases, a change in your diabetes medication may improve your blood glucose levels and, in turn, reduce your anxiety or depression. You might also want to discuss ways to help you stick more closely to your diabetes team's advice. Putting yourself in control of your problems is one of the best ways to beat anxiety and depression. On the other hand, feeling that your diabetes (or another problem) controls you is one of the most common causes of anxiety, depression and stress. Unfortunately, people living with depression or anxiety may be less motivated to stick to the lifestyle regimens and the treatments for diabetes. So, they may be more likely to develop complications.

Nevertheless, some people need additional help. If symptoms markedly affect your daily life, your doctor may suggest antidepressants or drugs to alleviate anxiety (anxiolytics). Don't dismiss antidepressants or anxiolytics out of hand. It's often difficult to plan the best way to overhaul your lifestyle to help control your diabetes in particular or tackle your life problems in general when you're carrying the burden imposed by depression or anxiety.

Although drugs can ease depression and anxiety, they don't cure the underlying problem. But antidepressants or anxiolytics may offer you a window of opportunity to improve control of your diabetes and deal with any other issues you face. Many people find that talking to a counsellor helps. Your GP may be able to recommend a local counsellor. Alternatively, you could contact the British Association for Counselling and Psychotherapy (see Useful addresses).

Counsellors and psychotherapists use a variety of 'talking therapies' to help you tackle your problems. One approach – cognitive behavioural therapy (CBT) – helps you identify the feelings, thoughts, behaviours and beliefs associated with diabetes. CBT will then help you identify which mental strategies are unhelpful and unrealistic and replace them with more appropriate approaches. In other words, CBT can help you face issues that you have avoided and try out new ways of behaving and reacting, which bolsters your defences against psychological problems, overcomes practical issues and helps improve your control of diabetes.

Depression and partners

Depressed people can feel they are living at the bottom of a deep well: even if they can see the light it seems faint and distant, and they feel that there is no way to climb out. Depression can mean that the person simply can't motivate themselves to seek help. A partner can encourage a depressed or anxious person with diabetes to seek help. But remember that any ladder you offer may seem rickety and unstable. You can help engender the confidence your partner needs to climb out. Emotional support shows you care and so boosts your partner's feeling of self-worth, both of which can help improve mental health.

Stress

Even if you don't suffer from full-blown clinical anxiety or depression, the pressure of living with diabetes may mean that you feel stressed out very easily. When you're stressed, your body pumps out hormones and other chemicals to get you ready to fight or run away. So, blood glucose levels rise to provide the body with the fuel it will need. This was fine when we faced a sabre-toothed cat or a rampaging rival tribe. The threat was relatively short-lived and we burnt the excess glucose off. However, it's less useful when we face an over-demanding boss, economic meltdown or the demands of living with a chronic disease. Such problems rarely offer the respite we need to relax. So, blood glucose levels remain high, which can undermine the control of your diabetes.

That's why you need to be particularly careful about monitoring your blood glucose levels, despite the other distractions, at times of particular stress, such as when you face redundancy, a bereavement or divorce. And, of course, your usual exercise and eating patterns can suffer at times of stress. You can work at keeping your stress levels down by using relaxation CDs, learning how to meditate, shiatsu and other types of massage, consulting a hypnotherapist or reading a few of the many books now available. Starting now can help bolster your defences when things get tough.

5

Treating diabetes with drugs

During the early years of the twentieth century, several researchers tried treating diabetes with extracts of the pancreas. Although these preparations reduced blood glucose levels, they were relatively impure. As a result, many people developed toxic reactions. Then in 1921, Canadian researchers, led by Fredrick Banting and Charles Best, prepared a relatively pure extract of insulin. The first patient they treated showed a disappointing response. But on 23 January 1922 they treated Leonard Thompson, a 14-year-old boy with T1DM who weighed just 65 lbs (29 kg), using an even more purified version. Leonard improved immediately.[1]

Their discovery transformed the care of diabetes – even for people with T2DM, once called non-insulin-dependent diabetes. A few people can control T2DM with diet and lifestyle changes alone. However, 80–90 per cent of people with T2DM need drugs to control their blood glucose levels.[2] And, over time, many people with T2DM take additional drugs, higher doses or insulin. One UK study found that over 6 years, around 53 per cent of people taking a type of tablet that reduces glucose called a sulphonylurea (page 59) starting using insulin.[3] Furthermore, because the body is less sensitive to insulin and because they tend to be heavier, people with T2DM often need a higher dose of insulin than those with T1DM.[2]

The search for tablets for diabetes

Nevertheless, in the early years at least, many people with T2DM show blood glucose levels that are dangerously high, but not sufficiently raised to warrant insulin. This prompted a search for oral drugs for diabetes. And one clue resided in Europe's herbal heritage.

Traditional healers have used goat's rue, also known as French lilac (*Galega officinalis*) as a diabetes treatment since at least the Middle Ages (for more on herbal treatments, see Chapter 10). In the 1920s, researchers discovered that a chemical in goat's rue, called guanidine, reduced blood sugar levels. Chemists altered guanidine's chemical structure to boost the blood glucose-lowering effect while reducing the risk of side effects. However, the result – a drug called synthalin – still caused a range of serious side effects, including nausea, diarrhoea and liver damage.[4]

People with diabetes had to wait until the 1950s for effective and relatively safe oral drugs,[4] when researchers found that a type of antibiotic called a sulphonamide lowered blood glucose. This lead to the development of a group of antidiabetic drugs called the sulphonylureas. Metformin, also launched in the 1950s for diabetes, and sulphonylureas remain mainstays of T2DM treatment today.[2]

Since then, numerous new forms of insulin and other drugs that lower blood glucose levels (hypoglycaemics) have reached the market. However, diet and other lifestyle changes remain the foundation of treatment. A single approach alone is unlikely to optimally control your diabetes. But diet combined with drugs and other lifestyle changes can dramatically reduce your risk of developing distressing, debilitating and even deadly complications, and help you live as normal a life as possible.

There's not space to look at the advantages and disadvantages of each drug for diabetes in detail. In any case, the balance depends on your particular circumstances. You should discuss the best choice for you with your diabetes care team. The wide range of treatments that are now available mean that you should be able to find a drug or combination of medicines that's right for you.

Insulin

Initially, people with diabetes received an injection of insulin extracted from the pancreases of pigs, cows or both (see page 5). Pork (porcine) or beef (bovine) insulin is a foreign protein, so the body may mount an immune reaction against the insulin, in much the same way as it does against bacteria. In some cases, the antibodies can cause side effects or stop the insulin from working effectively. In the 1980s doctors started using genetically engineered human insulins, which the manufacturers claimed were less likely to carry infections and cause immune reactions than animal-derived insulins. Some people with diabetes felt that the warning

Table 6 Types of insulin and their differing effects on blood glucose

	Time to peak effect	Duration of effect
Rapidly acting insulin analogues	60–90 minutes	3 hours
Short-acting (regular) insulin	2–3 hours	4–6 hours
Intermediate-acting insulin	4–8 hours	10–16 hours (in some cases up to 20 hours)
Long-acting insulin	3–8 hours (if at all)	14–24 hours

Times are approximate guides only and may vary between different analogues and between patients.

Source: Adapted from Mazze[5]

symptoms of hypoglycaemia changed when they switched from animal to human insulin.[4] However, almost all people with diabetes in the UK now receive genetically engineered human insulins.

Meanwhile, researchers were trying to develop insulins with durations of effect that more closely mimicked the release by the pancreas. For example, in the 1930s researchers found that a fish protein, called protamine, slowed insulin absorption. Other scientists discovered that mixing insulin with zinc also slowed absorption.[2]

More recently, pharmaceutical companies have created human insulins with a range of durations of action by changing the gene that encodes the protein (page 5). Changing the gene alters the chain of amino acids that make up insulin. Change too many amino acids and insulin won't work. But altering a few amino acids can change the protein's biological properties while retaining the activity on blood glucose levels.

For example, using a gene that switches two amino acids in the human chain creates an insulin analogue called lispro, which is absorbed more quickly than normal insulin. Lispro's effect on blood glucose levels peaks sooner and is shorter lived than that produced by normal insulin. Changing other amino acids can produce analogues with a much longer duration of effect.[5] Doctors now classify insulin into four types based on their duration of effect (Table 6).

This choice allows people with diabetes to match their insulin use to their lifestyle. For example:

- Some people take a 'bolus' of short-acting insulin with meals – which don't need be at regular times – and snacks, underpinned with a 'basal' long-acting insulin once or twice a day.
- Other people with diabetes inject a mix of rapid- or short-acting and intermediate-acting insulin at least twice a day, then eat meals at specific times each day, with snacks in between and activity at set times.[5]

Your diabetes team will help you decide which combination is right for you. But you need to make sure you know when to inject your insulin. For example:

- Short-acting insulins reduce your need to snack and help prevent hypos. However, the benefits are short-lived. So you need to inject some short-acting insulins about 15–20 minutes before a meal to mimic the normal production of insulin.
- You need to inject regular insulin between 30 and 40 minutes before eating.
- Immediate-release insulin acts for longer, but using too high a dose before the evening meal can trigger nocturnal hypos.[5]

However, these timings are generalizations. The timings for you depend on the specific product you use and the way your body responds. Your diabetes care team will tell you how best to use your insulin. So make sure you fully understand your treatment regimen, monitor your blood glucose levels and ask if you have any concerns.

Why is insulin injected?

Insulin is a protein – like a steak. So, if you swallowed insulin your body would digest the drug just as it digests a steak. Injecting insulin bypasses the digestion. But scientists have long sought an alternative to sometimes painful injections. Indeed, a drug company launched inhaled insulin in 2006. Users absorbed the protein across the lung when they breathed in. However, inhaled insulin was expensive, the product was not a commercial success and the company withdrew it about a year after launch. Despite this, many drug companies are searching for ways to deliver insulin without a jab and some alternatives may become available in the next few years. Researchers are even trying to protect insulin from digestion, raising the prospect of insulin tablets, although it will probably be several years before these become an established part of treatment.

Other drugs for diabetes

Most people with T2DM produce some insulin, although not enough to meet their needs. So, people with T2DM can take one or more drugs that boost the activity of the insulin that is still produced by their pancreas. Again, each of these drugs has advantages and disadvantages, and all are additions to, rather than replacements for, a healthy diet and lifestyle.

Metformin

Metformin, first used for diabetes in the 1950s, decreases glucose production by the liver and increases uptake by cells. This means that metformin acts only when the pancreas produces at least some insulin. Metformin doesn't directly increase insulin production. So there's almost no risk of hypoglycaemia when metformin is used alone.[2]

Metformin is especially useful in overweight people with T2DM. Indeed, many people lose weight during treatment with metformin. However, doctors should prescribe metformin only when diet has failed to reduce weight and blood glucose levels in an overweight person. Furthermore, around 10 per cent of people don't respond to metformin. Another 5–10 per cent will need to add at least one other drug to metformin.[2] So, if metformin alone does not adequately reduce blood glucose levels, doctors add another drug with a complementary mechanism of action, such as a sulphonylurea, pioglitazone, acarbose or a drug targeting the incretin pathway (see below).

Up to 30 per cent of people experience side effects with metformin, most commonly nausea, abdominal discomfort, diarrhoea and other gastrointestinal symptoms. However, these side effects usually improve with time. A few people absorb less vitamin B_{12} – a healthy diet will help (see page 111). Occasionally, people taking metformin develop a condition called lactic acidosis,[2] where a by-product of metabolism called lactic acid builds up in the bloodstream, causing nausea and weakness.

Sulphonylureas

Sulphonylureas (also called sulfonylureas or insulin secretagogues) increase insulin secretion from the pancreas. So, as with metformin, sulphonylureas (such as glibenclamide, gliclazide and tolbutamide) work only when some active beta cells remain. During long-term treatment, sulphonylureas seem to increase cells' insulin sensitivity. Doctors tend to use sulphonylureas for people with T2DM who:

- are not overweight – people taking sulphonylureas typically gain between 1 and 4 kg in the first 6 months of treatment;[6]
- are unable to take metformin because they develop side effects;
- have other conditions (such as some people with kidney disease) that preclude metformin's use.

As a rule, as sulphonylureas increase insulin secretion, the class is more likely than other non-insulin treatments for T2DM to cause hypoglycaemia. Indeed, sulphonylurea-related hypoglycaemia may last several hours and need treatment in hospital. Eating regularly also seems to reduce the risk. Furthermore, sulphonylureas differ in their propensity to cause hypoglycaemia. Glibenclamide, for example, has a longer duration of action and a higher risk of hypoglycaemia than gliclazide and tolbutamide. Nevertheless, hypoglycaemia usually indicates the dose of sulphonylurea is too high. So if you experience symptoms of hypoglycaemia (page 39) when taking a sulphonylurea you should see your diabetes nurse or GP.

Nateglinide and repaglinide

Nateglinide and repaglinide stimulate insulin release from the pancreas. Both drugs have a rapid onset and short duration of action on blood glucose levels. So, you take nateglinide and repaglinide shortly before each main meal and they are generally used in addition to metformin. However, people may take repaglinide alone if they are not overweight or cannot take metformin.

Pioglitazone

Pioglitazone (which belongs to a group of drugs called thiazolidinediones) reduces insulin resistance. Pioglitazone can be used alone or combined with metformin or a sulphonylurea. Such combinations increase insulin production and enhance cells' responsiveness. So, a doctor may suggest:

- adding pioglitazone to metformin rather than a sulphonylurea if the latter triggers hypos, or

- combining pioglitazone with both metformin and a sulphonylurea if blood glucose doesn't respond adequately to the combination of the latter two drugs.

However, if metformin and a sulfonylurea don't reduce your blood glucose levels sufficiently, your pancreas may be producing inadequate amounts of insulin. In some cases, using insulin may be a better choice than introducing pioglitazone. Your diabetes team can help you decide which is right for you.

A doctor or nurse will check that your HbA_{1c} concentration has declined by at least 0.5 per cent within 6 months of starting pioglitazone. If not, the diabetes team will probably advise that you stop pioglitazone and suggest an alternative.

Several other thiazolidinediones – also called 'glitazones' – were withdrawn after concerns about safety. Pioglitazone seems to increase the risk of heart failure when combined with insulin, especially in people who have certain risk factors, such as surviving a previous heart attack. So, your doctor may monitor you for signs of heart failure. You may also gain weight – typically between 1 and 4 kg during the first 6–12 months' treatment with thiazolidinediones.[2]

Pioglitazone also seems to be associated with an increased risk (between 12 and 33 per cent) of bladder cancer. Nevertheless, provided your blood glucose levels respond, the organization that regulates medicines in Europe believes that pioglitazone's benefits outweigh the risks. However, if you see blood in your urine, experience pain during urination or need to pass water urgently while taking pioglitazone, you should see your doctor speedily.

GLP-1 mimetic

As we saw in Chapter 1, hormones called incretins released by the gastrointestinal tract stimulate the pancreas to produce insulin. One of these hormones – called GLP-1 – has several key actions. It:

- stimulates insulin production
- increases the number of beta cells
- slows the speed at which food moves through the gut
- reduces appetite.

However, enzymes – most importantly one called DPP-4 (dipeptidyl peptidase 4) – break GLP-1 down within a few minutes.[4,6] This rapid degradation means that GLP-1 doesn't remain in the circulation long enough to treat T2DM.

A lizard in the Arizona desert held the answer. The venomous saliva of the Gila monster *(Heloderma suspectum)* contains a protein, called exendin-4, that stimulates insulin release.[6] The amino acid sequence (page 5) of about half of exendin-4 is identical to human GLP-1. And that's enough of a similarity to reduce blood sugar levels in humans, but different enough to resist DPP-4 and the other enzymes that break down GLP-1. So exendin-4 reduces blood glucose levels for a lot longer than GLP-1.

A drug company modified exendin-4 to produce a medicine called exenatide, which lowers blood glucose for 12 hours. Like insulin, digestion would break down exenatide, which is a protein. So, people with diabetes inject exenatide twice a day. A more recent version of the drug allows injection just once a week.[4]

More recently, another GLP-1 mimetic called liraglutide reached the market. T2DM patients inject liraglutide once a day. Both exenatide and liraglutide increase insulin secretion, suppress glucagon release and slow the speed at which food moves through the gut. Unlike some other drugs for diabetes, exenatide and liraglutide do not seem to increase weight. Indeed, some overweight people lose weight while taking exenatide or liraglutide.

The National Institute for Health and Clinical Excellence (NICE) recommends that treatment with GLP-1 mimetics continues only if patients benefit, such as showing a decline in HbA_{1c} of at least 1 per cent and a weight loss of at least 3 per cent within 6 months of starting exenatide or liraglutide. Doctors tend to use liraglutide and exenatide when blood glucose remains high in people taking combinations of two other drugs (e.g. metformin and a sulphonylurea) or when they can't take other treatments because of side effects or other diseases.

DPP-4 inhibitors

As mentioned above, an enzyme called DPP-4 breaks down the incretin GLP-1 within a few minutes. So scientists developed another group of drugs (which includes saxagliptin, sitagliptin and vildagliptin) that inhibit DPP-4. The resulting rise in incretin levels increases insulin secretion and lowers glucagon secretion. DPP-4 inhibitors are used alongside metformin or another glucose-lowering drug. Treatment generally continues only if HbA$_{1c}$ declines by at least 0.5 per cent within 6 months of starting treatment.

NICE suggests adding a DPP-4 inhibitor to metformin instead of a sulphonylurea when control of blood glucose remains or becomes inadequate (HbA$_{1c}$ at least 6.5 per cent; 48 mmol/mol) and if:

- hypoglycaemia poses a particular risk, such as in older people and people working at heights or with heavy machinery, or
- the person can't take a sulphonylurea.

Acarbose

Acarbose delays the digestion and absorption of starch and sucrose. As a result, acarbose slightly reduces blood glucose. Doctors tend to use acarbose when patients can't take other oral hypoglycaemics. Some people experience flatulence while taking acarbose, although this side effect tends to decrease with time.

6

Treating diabetes by changing your lifestyle

Modern medicines for diabetes are remarkably effective and relatively safe. Unfortunately, there's no magic bullet to treat diabetes. No single drug or combination of medicines allows you to eat what you want, when you want, with impunity, while avoiding complications. No single, simple lifestyle change reverses the damage wrought by chronically high blood glucose levels or guarantees that people with prediabetes won't develop T2DM. And all drugs have side effects and are unsuitable for some people.

So, most people need to combine drugs and lifestyle changes to control their diabetes. This chapter looks at some ways you can change your lifestyle – in addition to eating a healthy, balanced diet – to reduce your risk of developing T2DM, improve control of blood glucose levels and help prevent diabetic complications.

Losing weight

As we have seen, being overweight is the main risk factor for T2DM. And some drugs for diabetes can cause weight gain. So, NICE suggests that overweight people with T2DM should aim to lose 5–10 per cent of their body weight. However, if you simply can't manage to lose and keep off this much, even less marked weight loss may still boost your health and help you control your blood glucose levels. Indeed, losing weight, especially abdominal fat, improves cells' sensitivity to insulin. Shedding a few pounds also reduces levels of unhealthy fats circulating around your body and lowers blood pressure, which cuts your risk of complications, such as heart disease and strokes.

Eating 500–1,000 fewer calories each day can reduce body weight (assuming your BMI is stable) by between 0.5 and 1.0 kg each week.[1] But you'll need to keep eating healthily to ensure you keep the weight off. And if you have a medical condition (including diabetes) you should get the green light from your doctor before you embark on a weight loss programme. You may need to consult your dietician to find the best weight loss programme for you.

How to lose weight – and keep the pounds off

Unfortunately, losing weight is not easy – whatever the latest fad diets would have you believe. After all, millions of years of evolution drive us to consume food in times of feast to help us survive during times of famine. And you can't stop eating as you can quit smoking. However, the following tips may help:

- Set yourself a realistic target. Steadily losing around a pound or two a week reduces your chances of putting it back on again.
- Your exercise programme and the diet will help you lose weight. So, try to stick to them.
- Keep a food diary (page 74) and record everything you eat and drink for a couple of weeks. It's often easy to see where you inadvertently pile on the extra calories: the odd biscuit here, the extra glass of wine or full-fat latte there. It all adds up.
- Think about how you tried to lose weight in the past. What techniques and diets worked for you? Which failed to make a difference or were you unable to stick to?
- Tightly controlling your blood glucose levels also helps. Snacking can prevent hypoglycaemia, but can encourage weight gain.[2]
- To lose weight the healthy way you need to choose foods that keep you feeling full for longer. This means, for example, eating complex carbohydrates that slowly release their glucose rather than simple sugars (page 78). The slow trickle of glucose from complex carbohydrates into your bloodstream keeps you feeling full – it also helps you control your blood sugar levels.
- Set specific goals. Don't say that you want to lose weight: rather, resolve to lose, say, 2 stone (13 kg).
- Don't let a slip-up derail your diet. Try to identify why you indulged – what were the triggers? A particular occasion? Do you comfort eat? Are you veering towards hypos more frequently? Once you know why you slipped you can develop strategies to stop the problem in the future.

Setting a target weight

It's important to consider your height when setting your target weight, which is why doctors use BMI (page 18). Furthermore, the same volume of muscle weighs more than fat. So, people who frequently engage in challenging workouts, enjoy physically demanding sports or have strenuous jobs are likely to carry a lot of muscle on their bodies and may weigh more than a person of the same height but with comparatively little muscle. You can ask your doctor to measure your body fat, which, used alongside BMI, can help check whether you're a healthy weight and help set your target.

But there are times when you'll slacken the reins – such as when you're on holiday, celebrating or just bored with the diet and can't resist taking a few days off. Of course, slackening the reins also means, in some cases, that you may have to monitor your blood glucose more carefully and adjust the dose of insulin to match. Don't worry about these occasions too much. You're in this for the long term.

Avoid the crash...

In any case, no matter how overweight you are, it's not wise to lose weight too quickly. People who embark on a crash diet also inevitably feel deprived at some point. It's a normal reaction, but can lead to sudden irresistible urges to binge on junk food such as chocolate, cakes, pastries, burgers, pizzas and chips. We have already seen how the body's metabolism changes in reaction to starvation, such as switching to the amino acids in muscle as a source of glucose. Losing weight slowly – about between 0.5 and 1.0 kg each week – avoids triggering the starvation reaction and helps the changes in eating habits become second nature. In other words, slowly losing weight loss helps you to avoid swinging between weight loss and gain.

If you feel you need additional help and support think about joining a weight loss support group. You could ask your doctor or diabetes care team about groups in your area. Diabetes UK (see Useful addresses) also offers advice and support about weight management. If all this fails, try talking to your GP. A growing number of medicines may help kick-start your weight loss, though none is a magic cure.

Exercise

Glucose fuels your body's activities. The more you exercise the more fuel you need. So, physical activity lowers blood glucose levels. Therefore, it's important to be as active as possible. Weight-bearing activity increases mobility, strength and stamina, and helps protect against osteoporosis (thinning of the bones). Combining a healthy balanced diet with regular moderate exercise is more effective at controlling your blood glucose levels, reducing your risk of complications and becoming healthier than either one alone.

For example, exercise conditions the heart and cardiovascular system, greatly reducing your chances of developing hypertension, heart attacks, stroke and other complications. Your stamina will improve. Exercise also aids weight loss and helps you maintain your ideal weight. Regular exercise alone for 3 weeks reduces abdominal fat by approximately 20 per cent and weight by an average of 2.2 kg. In addition, exercise strengthens your immune system, combats stress and promotes sleep. So, it's no wonder that many people find exercise improves self-esteem.

How much exercise do I need?

Ideally, you should aim to be moderately active for at least 30 minutes on at least 5 days – and ideally every day – a week. It doesn't all have to be in one go. You can exercise for 15 minutes twice a day for example. You should aim to exercise until you are breathing harder than usual, but not so hard that you can't hold a conversation. You should feel that your heart is beating faster than usual and you've begun to sweat. However, if you experience chest pain stop exercising and see your doctor.

You should start slowly and build up your time as you feel able. However, if you are using insulin or are taking some another anti-diabetic drugs, you need to carefully monitor your blood sugar level to ensure that the exercise doesn't trigger a hypo. Ask your diabetes team if you're uncertain what to do.

Make exercise part of everyday life

You need to make exercise part of your everyday life. If you've been exercising regularly for a year, you'll lose about half your cardiovascular fitness in just 3 months if you stop. So, find a type of exercise that suits you and fits into your lifestyle. If you're not naturally a water baby or the pool is some distance from home or work you may be more likely to quit an exercise programme based on swimming. The following are relatively easy to fit in to a busy life.

Walking

Walking gives a fantastic whole-body workout. But to get the most benefit make sure you walk for about 30 minutes four or five times a week. Unfortunately, walking outdoors is not always practical. So, an electric treadmill can be an excellent investment, giving you the freedom to walk whenever you wish, whatever the weather. Some people consider treadmill walking monotonous and artificial. So, try reading, watching television or listen to your favourite music or podcasts – the miles can fly by. The American Heart Association suggests taking at least 10,000 steps a day. You could use a pedometer to ensure you walk far enough.

If you are very out of condition you may just want to walk to the nearest lamp-post and back on your first day. On the second and third days you should try to repeat that. On the fourth day you could try walking to the second lamp-post, on the fifth and sixth days to repeat that, on the seventh to the third lamp-post, on the ninth and tenth to repeat that and so on. For most people, walking is the easiest and most convenient aerobic activity. You may surprise yourself at how far you can walk after increasing the distance over several weeks.

Swimming

Swimming is a great exercise with a lower risk of injury than most other aerobic activities. Swimming works all the major muscles in the body without causing undue stress on the bones and encourages deeper breathing and increased oxygen intake.

If you get tired of swimming laps or aren't up to that, try simple kicking, treading water, slow running through the water or jumping on the spot. Be careful not to overdo it. Try to swim once or twice a week, gradually building up your swimming time to an hour-long session. However, as with any exercise, if you have another condition, in particular heart disease, speak to your doctor before swimming.

Cycling

Cycling using an exercise bike or outdoors provides an excellent cardiovascular workout. Diabetes and other health problems permitting, start by pedalling slowly, gradually building momentum. Limit your sessions to 2 or 3 minutes at first. You can then gradually build up to 20–30 minutes.

Participation sports

Participation sports are great for keeping fit, boosting your body's metabolic processes and meeting new people. Ask your sports centre, adult education centre or library about your local clubs for tennis, badminton, squash, football, rugby, netball, t'ai chi, dance classes and so on. There is usually a great choice of clubs in your local area and you'll soon find something that suits you.

Tips for being more active

As well as taking regular exercise, look for opportunities in your everyday life to become more active, such as:

- Walk to the local shops instead of taking the car.
- Ride a bike to work instead of travelling by car.
- Park further away, say a 15-minute walk, from your place of work.
- If you take the bus, get off one or two stops early and walk the remaining distance.
- Use the stairs instead of the lift.
- Clean the house regularly.
- Instead of using a carwash, clean the car by hand.
- Take up gardening – growing your own vegetables is also a great way to boost your consumption; they taste better as well.
- Walking to and from school gives the kids that important added exercise, and may help cut their risk of developing diabetes.

A word of warning

If you have arthritis, diabetic neuropathy or another condition that limits your mobility, ask for a referral to your local physiotherapy department. Physiotherapists can suggest the best exercise for your particular case. For example, some people with lower limb neuropathy, arthritis or other health problems find that they walk further on the treadmill's continuous level setting than on the variable terrain outdoors. So discuss your exercise programme with your doctor or diabetes care team.

Quit smoking

Nicotine, the addictive chemical in tobacco, and the plant's scientific name (*Nicotiana tabacum*) 'honour' Jean Nicot de Villemain (1530–1600), the French ambassador to Portugal who introduced tobacco to Parisian society when he returned from Lisbon in 1561. Tobacco rapidly became fashionable. But today smoking is increasingly socially unacceptable – just look at the huddles of smokers outside offices, pubs and restaurants. During the 1940s, around 70 per cent of men and 40 per cent of women smoked. According to government statistics, in 2009 22 per cent of men and 20 per cent of women in England smoked. That's a welcome decline. But about 8.8 million people still smoke.

Around half of those who don't quit smoking die prematurely. Indeed, during 2008 more than 80,000 people died prematurely in England from smoking-related diseases. For example:

- Smokers are roughly twice as likely to die from cancer as non-smokers.
- Smoking increases the likelihood of having a stroke up to threefold.
- Smoking underlies one-fifth of deaths among middle-aged people.
- Smoking causes around half of all cases of heart disease.
- Kidney damage is more common and, once nephropathy develops, worsens more quickly in people with diabetes who smoke compared with non-smokers.[3]
- Nerve damage is more common and worsens more quickly in people with diabetes who smoke compared with non-smokers.[3]

In other words, smoking further increases the risk of heart disease and stroke in people with diabetes, who are already especially likely to develop these conditions. Smoking can make breathing difficult, so your ability to exercise declines. And smoking can exacerbate some diabetic complications.

On the other hand, quitting reduces your likelihood of developing most smoking-related diseases. According to the

Department of Health, a lifelong smoker dies, on average, around 10 years sooner than they otherwise would. A person who stops smoking at 30 or 40 years of age gains, on average, 10 and 9 years of life respectively. Even a 60-year-old gains 3 years of life by quitting.

The dangers to your family

If the benefits to your health are not enough to make you quit, think of the harm you're doing to your loved ones. Second-hand smoke contains more than 4,000 chemicals, including over 50 carcinogens. This chemical cocktail increases the risk of serious diseases – including lung cancer, heart disease, asthma and sudden infant death syndrome – in people who inhale second-hand smoke. For example, the risks that a woman who has never smoked will develop lung cancer and heart disease are 24 and 30 per cent greater respectively, if she lives with a smoker.

Making quitting easier

Fewer than 1 in every 30 smokers manages to quit annually, and more than half of these relapse within a year. And ideally you need to quit, not cut down. People who reduce cigarette consumption usually inhale more deeply to get the same amount of nicotine. Nevertheless, cutting back seems to increase the likelihood that you'll eventually quit by, in some studies, 70 per cent compared with those who never cut back. In other words, reduction can take you a large step towards kicking the habit. But don't stop there.

Withdrawal symptoms when you stop smoking can leave you irritable, restless and anxious as well as experiencing insomnia and craving a cigarette, but usually abate over 2 weeks or so. Meanwhile, nicotine replacement therapy can alleviate this, and increases quit rates by between 50 and 100 per cent. Nicotine patches reduce withdrawal symptoms but have a relatively slow onset of action. Nicotine chewing gum, lozenges, inhalers and nasal spray act more quickly. Talk to your pharmacist or GP to find the right combination for you. If you still find quitting tough, doctors can prescribe other treatments. But there's no quick fix. You'll still need to be committed to quitting.

You can get a free 'quit smoking' support pack from the NHS Smoking Helpline (see Useful addresses). The website includes inspirational video clips, a stop smoking guide, an addiction test with advice for beating cravings, and an information sheet. Many areas also offer NHS antismoking clinics, often at a doctor's surgery, that offer advice, support and, when appropriate, a supply of nicotine replacement therapy. Other people find hypnotherapy helps them quit. If you would like to try this, ask your doctor for a recommendation or contact the British Association of Medical Hypnosis (see Useful addresses).

Tips to help you quit

Breaking tobacco's hold is tough. On some measures, nicotine is more addictive than heroin or cocaine. But, in addition to using nicotine replacement therapy, a few simple hints may make life easier:

- Set a quit date, when you will stop completely. Plan ahead: keep a diary of situations that tempt you to light up, such as coffee, meals, pubs or work breaks.
- Try to find something to take your mind off smoking. If you find yourself smoking when you get home in the evening, try a new hobby or exercise. Most people find that the craving for a cigarette usually only lasts a couple of minutes.
- Smoking is expensive. Keep a note of how much you save and spend at least some of it on something for yourself.
- Learn to deal with stress and hunger pangs. Military commanders from the Thirty Years War to the First World War encouraged smoking to blunt fear and hunger. You could try relaxation therapies to deal with stress. Try to avoid reaching for the sweet packet as a substitute for the nicotine. Following the healthy advice in this book, especially filling up on 'slow release' carbohydrates, should help stave off the hunger pangs. You may find you need to monitor your blood glucose especially carefully if quitting smoking changes your eating habits.

Nicotine is incredibly addictive and, not surprisingly, many people don't manage to quit first time. But if you relapse, try not to become too dispirited. Regard it as a temporary setback, set another quit date and try again. It's also worth trying to identify why you relapsed. Were you stressed out? If so, why? Was smoking linked to a particular time, place or event? Once you know why you slipped you can develop strategies to stop the problem in the future.

7

Diet and diabetes – the first steps

Ask many people what they mean by 'diet' and they will respond that it's eating in a way that means they will lose weight. We might hear someone say, 'I'm going on a low-fat diet so I can look good on the beach'. They may try a diet that supposedly helps a celebrity keep a chic figure. They may cut their calorie consumption gradually, crash diet, eat heroic amounts of grapefruit or cabbage soup, or stop eating carbohydrates. But in medical terms, 'diet' refers to the selection of foods you eat.

As mentioned on page 66, crash dieting rarely results in sustained weight loss. And you should never eliminate an essential food – such as wheat or dairy products – unless you're supervised by a dietician. It's easy to produce nutritional deficiencies. Such fads aren't a good idea for anyone, but may be especially dangerous for someone with diabetes. Eating large amounts of fruit can cause a marked rise in your blood glucose level, for example. A diet that includes disproportionate amounts of protein can result in hypos and even ketoacidosis.

Diabetic foods: an outdated term

Diabetic foods were a mainstay on chemist and supermarket shelves in the 1960s and early 1970s, when diabetes specialists suggested eating sugar-free, low-carbohydrate diets. Today, however, the term 'diabetic food' is increasingly obsolete. Indeed, in 2007 the Food Standards Agency and Diabetes UK issued a joint statement calling for an end to 'diabetic food' and 'suitable for diabetics' on food labels. Nevertheless, many people with diabetes and their families continue to believe that diabetic foods are wiser choices than conventional foods. Unfortunately, diabetic foods tend to be more expensive than conventional, sugar-free and reduced-sugar versions. And sweets, biscuits and similar foods often include the 'diabetic food' label, which could undermine healthy eating messages. As we'll see in the next chapter, everyone – diabetic or not – should eat foods and drinks containing added sugars sparingly.

73

Overhauling your diet, even for the better, can seem daunting. But many people find that it takes only a month or so of eating (or not eating) a food that's a mainstay of your diet for it to become a habit. Even people with a sweet tooth who cut back on sugar soon find themselves accustomed to the new taste and begin to dislike sweetened drinks. The same applies when you switch full-fat for skimmed milk. Some people soon find that they dislike the taste of full-fat milk. So, it's often easier than you may imagine to stick to a new diet. The improvements in your health and appearance then make it easier to keep following a healthy diet.

Stick to a routine

Some people dislike routine, or find it difficult to fit into their hectic lives. But following a daily routine helps you:

- take your drugs as agreed with your doctor;
- avoid slipping into hyperglycaemia or suffering a hypo;
- make the changes to your diet and lifestyle that cut the chances of diabetic complications.

So, you should take your medications at roughly the same time every day. You should test your blood glucose levels when advised to by your GP or diabetes team. And make time for routine exercise, such as a daily walk and your exercise classes and clubs. Choosing an activity you enjoy and that is local to you makes it easier to stick with a regular exercise programme. Finally, a healthy diet soon becomes part of your everyday life. So how should you start?

Keep a food diary

Keeping a daily record of everything you eat and drink, and when, is an excellent way of identifying problems with your current diet – such as where those hidden calories creep in (see Table 7). You can also enter your blood glucose readings to see if there is any link between your diet and, for example, low levels.

You may think you know how much junk food, vegetables, sugar and alcohol you consume. But it's amazing how often our guesses are wrong. For example, it's easy to forget the food you nibble on while cooking, those extra slices of bread and butter you eat to fill

Table 7 Example of a food diary

Time	Food (how cooked and where eaten)	Serving size	Exercise	Blood glucose reading	Insulin type, dose and time	Symptoms

up on after a meal, or the snacks you eat when your blood glucose levels dip. Parents often pick at their children's leftovers. When you're out with friends you may underestimate how much alcohol you drink. And many people think they eat more fruit and vegetables than they do.

One study, for example, found that, on average, we underestimate the amount of calories we eat by one-fifth, whether we use a diary or just try to remember. This suggests that people aren't completing the diary properly. The fatter you are, the more you underestimate your consumption.[1] And according to a report published by Alcohol Concern in 2009, the average adult drinker underestimates his or her consumption by the equivalent of a bottle of wine each week (a 750 ml bottle of 12 per cent wine contains 9 units).

Keeping a food diary can take considerable commitment. But if you have diabetes and are taking insulin or some other antidiabetic drugs you need to try to indentify which foods have a disproportionate effect on your blood glucose levels and which you can continue to enjoy. The food diary will also give a clearer picture of how much, and what, you eat and drink in a day. If you have prediabetes or are controlling T2DM with lifestyle changes alone, the food diary will reveal your bad habits and identify changes that could make a difference.

You'll need a dedicated notebook (or use a computer or smartphone app). Some people begin by recording their snacks and drinks – all of them – and how many spoonfuls of sugar they take in their tea and coffee for a few days. This eases them into the routine of note-making. When you are used to picking up your pen after eating, you can graduate to listing all the foodstuffs you tuck away each mealtime.

When you have kept your food diary for a couple of weeks your pattern of eating habits should be clear, as should the effects of your current food choices on your blood glucose levels. You've made a good start at taking your health into your own hands, but now you need to know how to improve your diet – we'll look at the details in the next couple of chapters.

As you improve your diet, keep up with the food diary and blood glucose testing. In time, you'll be able to look back to see just how far you've come in changing your diet and taking control of your diabetes. It's often easy to forget how unhealthy your diet was.

Changing negative thinking

Changing your lifestyle, not to mention living with a serious chronic disease, is often difficult. So, it's easy to slip into self-defeating, negative self-talk such as 'I'll never do this', 'I've got no willpower' and 'It's too hard to change'. But you *can* change a negative attitude into a more positive one. You may need to:

- recognize negative, defeatist self-talk.
- acknowledge that you can recognize and change negative thought patterns.
- realize that changing to positive thinking takes a little patience and determination.
- understand that positive thinking can make a great difference, in not just your diet, but all areas of your life.
- learn to 'assert' your diet in difficult situations – which may mean, for example, not keeping pace with friends' drinking or making healthy choices when around the family dinner table.

So how do you change negative into positive self-talk? You could repeat certain phrases out loud at least twice a day, perhaps as you stand in front of a mirror. At first this may feel a little artificial. But in time you should come to believe what you are saying. You could affirm, for example:

- 'My new diet will help me to control my diabetes.'
- 'Healthy eating will give me more energy and improve my health.'
- 'Healthy eating will help to prevent diabetes-related complications.'

- 'My diet will help me control my diabetes.'
- 'The diet will make me feel good about myself.'
- 'I enjoy exercise.'
- 'I'm an intelligent person and I can do this.'
- 'I don't need to feel alone because everyone's behind me.'
- If you are overweight, you could repeat to yourself 'The diet will help me to lose weight'.

Congratulate yourself each time you get through a day without eating something that's bad for you, such as a cake, alcohol or fat-laden snack. At the end of each successful week, reward yourself by buying a treat or going out to the cinema or theatre. Some people find that speaking to a counsellor, therapist or a hypnotherapist can give them the self-confidence and practical advice that they need to improve their diet and health.

Don't eat too fast

Your brain takes between 10 and 15 minutes to recognize that you have eaten enough and send signals to your body that you're full. That's one reason why it's a good idea not to eat too quickly. In just a few minutes you could stuff in more food than your body requires! The excess is then stored in fat cells. And eating fast can contribute to heartburn and indigestion. So eat slowly. Take your time and enjoy your food – even if it is just a sandwich at your desk or a baked potato for lunch when the rest of the family is out of the house.

8

Controlling carbs

Doctors' attitudes to carbohydrates in diabetes have changed dramatically over the years. Before insulin's introduction, doctors suggested that people with diabetes should cut carbohydrate consumption to starvation levels. As late as the early 1970s, doctors advocated treating diabetes with sugar-free, low-carbohydrate diets. However, attitudes began to shift as a growing body of scientific evidence showed that restricting carbohydrates – particularly complex carbohydrates, such as fibre and starch – did not improve diabetes control. Indeed, limiting complex carbohydrates encouraged people to eat energy-dense foods (e.g. cakes, crisps and biscuits), many of which are high in fat. The resulting weight gain and increased fat levels could exacerbate diabetes' long-term complications, particularly heart disease. So, by the 1980s, health authorities in the UK and many other countries were advising people with diabetes to focus on restricting fat consumption and controlling calorie intake.

This chapter focuses on carbohydrates. However, remember that diabetes is not only a disease of abnormal glucose levels; it's also a disease of abnormal fats. And remember that focusing on carbohydrate could unbalance your food choices, so you also need to follow the advice in the next chapter to create a healthy, balanced diet.

What are carbohydrates?

There are, broadly, two main types of carbohydrate, both of which supply energy: complex carbohydrates and simple sugars.

- Complex starchy carbohydrates include rice, chapattis, yam, noodles, cereals, pasta, potatoes and bread.
- Simple sugars include caster, granulated and other table sugars, and fruit sugar (fructose). Apart from the sugar we sprinkle in tea and coffee, dairy foods (lactose), pies, pastries, biscuits and cakes all contain simple sugars.

Carbohydrates are long chains of sugars. Starch consists of long chains of glucose, for example. Sucrose (table sugar) contains glucose joined to fructose. Digestion breaks carbohydrates into single sugars, of which glucose is the most important.

So after we eat carbohydrates, blood glucose levels rise. But exactly to what extent and for how long depends on the type of carbohydrate and, to a lesser extent, the other components of our diet, such as the amount of protein and fat. For example, glucose levels rise within a few minutes of swallowing a drink laden with several teaspoons of sugar. But the body takes longer to convert a bowl of wholewheat pasta into glucose in the blood. In other words, complex carbohydrates have a much longer-lasting effect on blood glucose levels than simple sugars.

According to European guidelines for diabetes, you should eat no more than 50 g of free sugars a day.[1] Free sugar refers to sugars that manufacturers, cooks or consumers add while preparing food as well as the sugars naturally present in honey, syrups and fruit juices. However, much of the sugar in our diet is hidden, which is where glycaemic index and load can help.

Labelling sweet talk

Some food labels refer to monosaccharides and disaccharides – saccharide is the chemical term for sugar. The mono- and di- refers to the number of sugars – mono is one, di is two. So glucose is a monosaccharide. Sucrose is a disaccharide.

Glycaemic index and glycaemic load

The glycaemic index (GI) ranks foods based on their effect on blood glucose. Weight for weight, foods that contain large amounts of slowly absorbed carbohydrate produce a steady rise in blood glucose with a relatively low peak – a bit like a gentle hill. These foods have a lower GI rating. Foods containing high levels of simple sugars produce a more rapid rise and a higher peak in blood glucose – more like a mountain. These foods have a higher GI rating.

Specifically, scientists measure the effect on blood glucose levels over 2–3 hours produced by 50 g of the food being tested, such as a burger or a bowl of cereal. They compare the rise to that produced by 50 g of glucose or white bread, which scientists define as having a GI of 100.

This approach can discriminate the effect on blood glucose levels produced by different types of carbohydrate. For example, 50 g of bread does not have the same effect on blood glucose as 50 g of fruit, and both differ from 50 g of pasta. So, the GI for these foods differs. GI can also distinguish between types of the same food. Some breads that include whole grains have a lower GI than the same weight of wholemeal (where the whole grain is ground up) or white bread.

So, choosing slowly absorbed, low GI carbohydrates helps maintain relatively constant blood glucose levels:

- A low GI meal helps you avoid hypos. Indeed, the benefits can persist until the following meal, ironing out peaks and troughs in glucose throughout the day.
- Slow-acting carbohydrates reduce the marked peaks in blood glucose following a meal (the 'postprandial glucose concentration' in the jargon), which, Diabetes UK comments, may help prevent T2DM.
- Low GI foods also help you lose, or stay at a healthy, weight. The slow release of glucose means you feel fuller for longer. So, you're less likely to snack between meals. This helps you stick to a weight loss diet.
- Low GI diets seem to reduce the risk of heart disease and raise levels of healthy HDL-cholesterol (page 27).

Planning your daily meals around foods with a low GI (or low glycaemic load; see below) improves the glucose profile after you eat.[1] Table 8 shows some examples of low, medium and high GI foods. Obviously, this isn't a comprehensive list. So read the label, some of which now state if the food is low GI. You can buy books that include the GI values for a wider range of foods. You can also find lists on the internet including:

- <www.diabetes.org.uk/Guide-to-diabetes/Food_and_recipes/ The-Glycaemic-Index>
- <http://care.diabetesjournals.org/content/31/12/2281/suppl/ DC1>
- <www.glycemicindex.com>.

Table 8 Examples of low-, medium- and high-GI foods

Glycaemic index		Food
Low	Less than 55	Apples, oranges, pears, peaches
		Beans and lentils
		Pasta made from durum wheat, noodles
		Sweet potato (peeled and boiled)
		Sweetcorn
		Porridge, All-Bran, Special K, Sultana Bran
		Custard
		Wholegrain breads
		Some raw fruits
Medium	55–70	Honey, jam
		Shredded Wheat, Weetabix
		Ice cream
		New potatoes (peeled and boiled)
		White basmati rice (cooked)
		Pitta bread
		Couscous
High	70–100	Glucose (e.g. tablets)
		White and wholemeal bread
		Brown and white rice (cooked)
		Cornflakes
		Baked and mashed potatoes
		White bread
		Biscuits
		Sugary drinks

Source: Diabetes UK and Toeller[1]

Limitations of the GI

Although the GI can help you make healthy food choices, it also has some important limitations:

- Comparing a food with glucose rather than white bread can influence GI. One brand of toasted bread had a GI of 72 compared with white bread and 50 compared with glucose. So, the toast was high GI in one analysis and medium in the other.[1]

- A low GI diet isn't necessarily healthy. Ice cream is often medium GI. Chocolate is low or medium GI. But both are high in saturated fat. Crisps and chips become bloated with fat during cooking. So, the British Dietetic Association (BDA) points out, potato crisps are medium GI. A baked potato is high GI. But a baked potato is far better for you than fat- and salt-laden crisps.
- Eating sufficient fibre (page 95) can be difficult if you're eating a low-carbohydrate diet.[1] A high-fibre diet helps prevent constipation, aids weight loss, reduces cholesterol and cuts your risk of developing colon (bowel) cancer.
- GI and glycaemic load (see below) aren't fixed. For example, you need to be careful if you use international tables. Many food brands are international. However, the composition of the same brand may differ from country to country to meet the demands of the local palate and market. Furthermore, the GI of some foods seems to be increasing, partly as manufacturers try to make food preparation and cooking easier and quicker. The GI of porridge oats, for instance, can vary depending on the extent of refining.[1]

Finally, we don't eat single foods. We eat bread and butter. We eat 'meat and two veg' or pasta and sauce. A curry or stew can contain a large number of ingredients, including meat, vegetables and herbs. Fenugreek, for example, a mainstay of curry recipes, is one of several herbs that can lower blood glucose levels – see page 114. It's unlikely, however, that the low amounts in a typical curry have much of an effect.

The other parts of the meal can influence a food's GI. For example, fat and protein can hinder carbohydrate absorption. That's one reason why milk and dairy products have a low GI. So:

- The BDA notes that liberal dollops of sugar-rich jam means you digest low GI granary bread more quickly.
- Eating a sweet sponge after a meal slows the cake's digestion.
- Mashed potato is high GI – adding cheese reduces the GI, but increases the fat.
- A baked potato is high GI – adding tuna, baked beans or cheese makes the meal low GI.
- Even adding vinegar to chips lowers the GI.[1]

So, think about the meal overall, rather than focusing on a specific food.

The limitations of the GI are one reason nutritionists tend to emphasize a healthy, balanced – rather than a low-carbohydrate – diet. You need to think about the number of calories, fibre, vitamins and minerals and not get hung up on the GI, even if you find it helps as a guide. A state-registered dietician can give you individual advice on food choices.

Glycaemic load

Spaghetti is a low GI food. But eat a lot of spaghetti and your blood glucose levels will rise. And, as we have seen, GI uses 50 g of the food as the basis for the calculation. However, a typical serving of a food may not be exactly 50 g. A slice of bread may weigh 30 g, while a typical portion of frozen peas may be 80 g. Obviously, the portion size influences the amount of carbohydrate we eat and, therefore, the effect on blood sugar. Glycaemic load (GL) builds on the foundation of GI by also considering portion size. Again, GL splits into three groups:

- high: GL of 20 or more
- medium: GL 11 to 19
- low GL: 10 or less.

Not surprisingly, some sugar-packed sports drinks, as well as certain bagels and cakes, have GL over 20. On the other hand, almost all low GL foods have a low GI. But between these extremes the picture is a little more complex. A breakfast cereal, for example, could have a GI of 72. But the 30 g serving gives a GL of 18. This breakfast cereal is high GI, medium GL.[2]

Not surprisingly, GL can seem confusing – although books and internet lists can help. And as GL is a refined version of GI, but uses the same basic principle, many of the same criticisms apply. In particular, GL only tells you about the carbohydrate content and not whether the food is healthy. So, while, some people find GL easier to use than the GI, some health professionals may feel both are too complex and variable for everyday use.[2] So if you want to use GL or GI to guide your food choices and are unsure ask your diabetes team or a dietician.

Carbohydrate counting

Over the last few years, food labels have contained increasingly detailed information. This means you can use the information to count carbohydrates and adjust your dose of insulin appropriately. Many people with diabetes find that basing insulin doses on carbohydrate counting allows more flexible diets, while enhancing blood glucose control. Indeed, many structured education programmes (such as DAFNE; see page ix) teach carbohydrate counting.[3]

Basically, you look at the total carbohydrate in 100 g of the food. Don't use the 'of which sugars' value when carb counting. You use the total of sugar and starch. Then check the portion or serving size, which can be considerably less than you may expect to eat. That gives the carb count. But remember to check whether the amount is cooked or not, especially with pasta and rice meals.

You can use carb counts to ensure you keep your intake constant and to estimate how many grams of carbohydrate 1 unit of insulin will cover. You can count the grams of carbohydrate in the food you want to eat and divide by your carb factor. This tells you how many units of bolus insulin (page 57) you need to cover the meal. Your diabetes team can let you know more about carbohydrate counting and work out your carb factor.

Non-sugar sweeteners

Sugar comes in a wide range of forms (see box) and can creep into your diet in many ways. Manufacturers add sugar during food production. Your partner may add sugar when preparing a meal. And you may 'automatically' add sugar to your tea, coffee and food at the table. So, many people – and not just those with diabetes – use non-sugar sweeteners to help control their weight.

The many faces of sugar

Sugar comes in many forms including:

- sucrose (white table sugar), which is derived from sugar beet or cane sugar and sold in powder or granulated form
- brown sugar (such as muscovado and Demerara)
- icing sugar
- raw sugar, in the form of granulated crystals
- glucose – sometimes called dextrose
- honey, which contains glucose, maltose and sucrose.

Indeed, if you look at the label, many sugar-free and low-calorie foods and drinks replace sugar with one of the 'polyol' sweeteners, such as sorbitol, maltitol, xylitol, isomalt and mannitol. Polyols have fewer calories than sucrose: saving up to 40 calories from 20 g of sweetener according to the Food Standards Authority.

Furthermore, the body doesn't absorb all the carbohydrate from polyols. So polyols have less effect on blood glucose levels than sucrose. As a result, people may need less insulin when they eat polyol sweeteners.

Nevertheless, switching to polyols may not be enough on its own to improve blood glucose control or markedly reduce weight. Furthermore, excessive consumption of polyol sweeteners can produce diarrhoea and flatulence, especially in young children.

Try to wean yourself off sugar as much as possible. You could start by changing from soft drinks to mineral water, or gradually reduce the amount of sugar you add to tea and coffee. When you're preparing food, try fruit and fruit juice, which make excellent sweeteners. But you should consume fructose (natural fruit sugar) in moderation. Fructose may increase levels of both triglycerides (a harmful type of fat) and uric acid (a chemical linked to gout) in blood[1] and consuming large amounts can drive your blood sugar levels up.

Celebrations

If you're taking insulin or another antidiabetic drug you can switch sucrose-containing foods for other carbohydrates in your meal plan. But don't switch too often. You need to avoid excess calories and watch your blood glucose levels. Nevertheless, just because you're diabetic, that doesn't mean you have to miss out on birthday cakes, parties and Christmas celebrations.

If you generally eat a healthy diet, these occasional celebrations won't do you any long-term harm, although you may need to adjust your dose of insulin by, for example, carb counting. Indeed, around Christmas and other celebrations you need to watch your blood glucose levels especially carefully; mince pies and Christmas cake, for example, tend to be loaded with calories, fat and sugar. And meals often tend to be larger than usual. It's also easy to become distracted by family and friends – and eat more than you planned. But try not to eat too much and look around for healthier versions. Diabetes UK often suggests seasonal recipes.

You should make sure the meal includes plenty of fruit, vegetables and starchy carbohydrates. That's a good idea for everyone, not just those with diabetes. You could try offering vegetable crudités, olives and dried fruit as an alternative to high-fat snacks and chocolate. Finally, get off the sofa – even walking around the January sales helps.

Raised blood glucose level is the hallmark of diabetes. However, modern medicines combined with lifestyle changes and careful meal planning mean that most people can control blood glucose levels to avoid hypos and reduce the risk of debilitating complications. Nevertheless, focusing excessively on carbohydrates runs the risk of missing other essential nutrients. You need to eat a healthy, mixed diet to help reduce your likelihood of developing heart disease and other diabetic complications. In Chapter 9, we'll look at the other elements of a healthy diet.

9

Diet and diabetes – beyond carbs

Changes in carbohydrate consumption cause fluctuating blood glucose levels. But don't become too hung up on carbohydrates. A healthy, balanced diet that includes foods from all groups is essential to maintain and improve health for everyone, not just those who have diabetes.

Alcohol and soft drinks

Everyone needs to watch how much alcohol they consume. But people with diabetes who are susceptible to hypoglycaemia, such as those taking insulin or some other antidiabetic drugs, should be particularly careful. Alcohol lowers blood glucose levels (partly by reducing release from the liver) and the effect can last for hours. So while people with diabetes with stabilized blood glucose levels can enjoy social drinking, they must always be on their guard against hypos. If you're at risk of hypos your diabetes team will often agree a limit on your drinking with you. This may differ from the safe drinking levels outlined below.

Unfortunately, the symptoms of a hypo (such as staggering, passing out and confusion; see page 39) can resemble drunkenness. So, if your breath smells of alcohol, doctors may think that you're drunk and not treat your hypo. That's one reason why you should always carry diabetes ID (such as a bracelet, card or necklace) with you. If you don't have such ID, speak to your diabetes team or GP.

If you lose control of your drinking and you're feeling rough the morning after, check your blood glucose level to ensure that the headache, nausea, shaking and sweats *really* are the result of indulgence rather than a hypo. Try your best to eat some breakfast. But if you can't face food (or you are vomiting), drink as much fluid as you can, including some sugary drinks. And don't stop taking your insulin or other antidiabetic medication.

Carbohydrate in alcoholic drink

In brewing and winemaking, yeasts convert the sugar in grain or grapes to alcohol. However, alcoholic drinks contain widely different amounts of carbohydrate. Dry wines and spirits contain little or no carbohydrate. Beer, lager and cider contain moderate amounts. Alcopops, sweet sherry and wines, and port contain large amounts.[1]

Many people now plump for low-alcohol or alcohol-free lager. While this is great from a medical, public safety and addiction point of view, low-alcohol beers may be higher in sugar than the standard sort. On the other hand, some breweries market low-sugar (sometimes promoted as diabetic) brands. But these convert more of the sugar to alcohol. Just 1 pint of some low-sugar beers can send you over the drink–drive limit.

Drinking safely

So, if you want to drink:

- Stay within the safe drinking levels: Diabetes UK suggests no more than 3 units a day for men and a maximum of 2 units for women. However, any advice from your diabetes team overrides this recommendation. And make sure you have some drink-free days each week.
- Don't drink on an empty stomach. Have a meal before you go out or, if it's an aperitif, within half an hour of your first drink. If you can't eat beforehand, eat carbohydrate-containing snacks such as a sandwich, nuts or crisps throughout the time you're drinking.
- Make sure your family or friends know what to do if you have a hypo. Drinking may make you less aware of a hypo's warning signs and, as mentioned above, even doctors can confuse a hypo with drunkenness.
- Alternate alcoholic beverages and either water or sugar-free soft drinks. This slows your alcohol consumption and helps avoid dehydration.
- Even diluting alcohol with mixer drinks can still have dangers. A shandy made from beer or lager and lemonade, for instance, is still high in sugar. Use diet drinks and soda, or – even better – water, as a mixer with spirits.

- Alcohol's effects can persist for hours after you stop drinking. The liver removes about 1 unit of alcohol from your blood every hour. However, the rate varies markedly from person to person. This means that you're still at risk of a hypo several hours after you stop drinking. So, eat some food – even chips or a kebab, but ideally something healthier, such as cereals or toast – before going to bed to help avoid nocturnal hypos.

Fighting the fat

Some of us lament the end of going to work fuelled by a fry-up. In 1989 we ate on average 112 g of fat a day, the British Heart Foundation remarks. By 2008 our fat intake had declined to 83 g a day. Yet many of us still eat too much fat: one reason why the nation's waistbands are bulging and diabetes is increasingly common. Fat is the most concentrated source of energy in our diet – 1 g of fat provides 9 calories. So, reducing fat aids weight reduction and helps you avoid heart disease and strokes.

Fats slow the absorption of carbohydrates into the bloodstream, staving off hunger pangs and helping stabilize blood glucose levels. The fat in fish and chips, burgers and fries, and some Indian and Chinese takeaway meals can slow carbohydrate absorption, for example. Many low GI foods can be high in fat. So it's easy for a person with diabetes to eat too much fat.

A diet high in fat, especially from animal sources, boosts levels of cholesterol in your blood. The higher level of cholesterol increases your risk of atherosclerosis (see page 44) and, in turn, peripheral vascular disease, heart attacks and some strokes. But despite its bad press, cholesterol is essential. For example, cholesterol:

- is a key part of the membranes that surround every cell;
- helps form the insulation around many nerve fibres (myelin sheath) that ensure signals travel properly;
- forms the backbone of several hormones, including oestrogen, testosterone and progesterone.

But poor diets and a lack of exercise (which burns up fat) mean that many of us have too much of a good thing.

Types of fat

Broadly, foods contain two types of fat:

- Saturated fat comes mainly from animal sources, and is generally solid at room temperature.
- Unsaturated fat derives mainly from vegetables, nuts and seeds, and is usually liquid at room temperature. Olive, rapeseed, safflower and sunflower oils are all unsaturated fats. There are two main subtypes: monounsaturated and polyunsaturated. As we'll see, fish is especially high in a particularly beneficial type of polyunsaturated fat (page 92).

Controlling cholesterol

Few foods contain high levels of cholesterol: eggs, liver, kidneys and prawns are some notable exceptions. As a result, our diet accounts for only around one-third of the cholesterol in the body. So, the idea that you need to eat no more than three eggs a week is now outdated. Eggs are one of the most nutritious foods and also contain lecithin, which seems to reduce the amount of cholesterol the body absorbs. It's fine to go to work on an egg, as part of a balanced diet.

Rather than worrying about cholesterol, focus on saturated fat in meat, full-fat dairy products, cakes, biscuits, pastries and so on. The liver converts saturated fat into cholesterol. Eating foods rich in saturated fat also slows the rate at which your body removes cholesterol. However, the BDA notes that most people in the UK eat about 20 per cent more than the recommended levels for the general population (no more than 20 g and 30 g of saturated fat a day for women and men, respectively). Saturated fat, according to guidelines for diabetes in the USA, should account for no more than 7 per cent of your total energy. European guidelines suggest that oils that are rich in monounsaturated fat should account for 10–20 per cent of total energy. Overall, fat should make up less than 35 per cent of your calories.[2] So, most of us should try to eat less food high in saturated fat. The BDA points out that:

- High-fat foods contain more than 5 g of saturated fat per 100 g.
- Low-fat foods contain 1.5 g or less saturated fat per 100 g.

Table 9 Foods high in saturated fat and the low-fat alternative

	Avoid	*Low-fat alternative*
Snacks	Crisps/savoury snacks cooked in oil	Fresh or dried fruit, handful of nuts
Fats for cooking and spreading	Lard, dripping, ghee, cream and butter	Olive, sunflower, soya or rapeseed (blended vegetable) oils, margarines and spreads; store oils in a sealed container in a cool, dark place to prevent rancidity
Meat	Fatty products (sausages, burgers, pâté, salami, meat pies and pasties)	Lean cuts of meat and mince (check labels or ask the butcher); trim off fat Skinless chicken and turkey Vegetarian options (e.g. lentils, chickpeas and soya)
Fish	Deep fried (e.g. takeaway) fish and chips	Oily fish such as salmon, mackerel and sardines
Sauces	Creamy or cheesy sauces	Tomato or vegetable-based sauces
Dairy	Full-fat varieties	Skimmed (or at least semi-skimmed) milk, reduced-fat cheddar and low-fat yoghurt; Try grating cheese or using a strongly flavoured variety, which may mean you need to use less; Edam, Camembert, Brie, reduced fat cheddar and cottage cheese contain less fat than many full-fat hard cheeses such as standard cheddar, Stilton, Parmesan and cream cheese

Source: Adapted from British Dietetic Association

Table 9 suggests some ways you could cut your consumption of saturated fat. The cooking method makes a big difference to levels of fat. It's better to grill, steam or oven-bake food instead of frying. If you must fry something, cook using a small amount of olive oil at a low temperature. You could also try sautéing in a little water or tomato juice.

The trans fat danger

Look at the labels of some of the biscuits, cakes and spreads in your larder. Hopefully you won't have too many. If you do, perhaps it's time to spring-clean your food stores. Many contain trans fatty acids, which gram for gram increase heart disease risk more than saturated fats. Unfortunately, numerous foods, including cheese, cream, beef, lamb and mutton, contain trans fatty acids. Heating vegetable oils to fry foods also creates trans fatty acids: one reason why it's better to steam, bake or grill.

Furthermore, a widely used method in food production (hydrogenation) can convert vegetable oils into solids or semi-solids containing trans fats. Biscuits, pies and cakes as well as some margarines and other spreads often contain hydrogenated (or trans-unsaturated fats). So, look for foods labelled 'low in trans' or 'virtually trans-free', and check the ingredients. Foods containing hydrogenated fats or hydrogenated vegetable oils almost always include trans fatty acids. You could try spreads made from the oils of nuts and seeds (such as peanut butter and sunflower oil) instead of butter and margarine.

Fish and omega-3 fatty acids

Life inside the Arctic Circle is tough. Few plants survive. So the traditional diet of First Nation Arctic people consists almost entirely of fish, seal and other meats. In the 1970s, for example, Greenland Inuit people ate around 400 g of seafood a day.[3] Despite this meat-based diet, First Nation Arctic people seem to be less vulnerable to several diseases, including diabetes, heart disease, arthritis and asthma, than people in industrialized countries.

But, like all of us, they are what they eat. Traditional diets of First Nation Arctic people are high in fish and animals that, in turn, eat marine life. So, they eat large amounts of polyunsaturated fish oils. Certain fish oils (called omega-3 or n-3 fatty acids) appear to have several important health benefits, including:

- reducing inflammation;
- increasing levels of the healthy fat HDL;
- cutting triglyceride levels;
- lowering blood pressure;
- making blood less likely to clot;
- reducing the chance that an atherosclerotic plaque will burst (page 45).

As a result, eating oily fish helps lowers your risk of cardiovascular disease. For example:

- Heart attacks were ten times less common among Greenland Inuit than in people from Denmark. On average, Greenland Inuit people ate 14 g of omega-3 fatty acids a day, the Danes just 3 g.[3]
- Eating fish once or twice a week (or 30–60 g a day) reduces the risk of death from coronary disease by 30–60 per cent.[4]
- In people who have already suffered a heart attack, eating 200–400 g of fatty fish a week or taking a supplement containing 1 g per day omega-3 fatty acids reduces the risk of dying from heart disease by between 20 and 30 per cent. However, if you use insulin or another medicine to help control your diabetes it's important to speak to your diabetes team before starting supplements – see Chapter 10.[4]

Eating fish regularly has several other benefits. Oily fish, the BDA points out, keep your joints healthy. Omega-3 polyunsaturated fatty acids (PUFAs) are also important for memory, intellectual performance and seem to protect the eyes of experimental animals from damage from diabetes.

Your retina contains millions of light-sensitive 'photoreceptors': about 120 million rods, which are responsible for dark-adapted vision, and 6–7 million cones, which are sensitive to colour. In one study, diabetes reduced rod function in rats by one-third. A diet rich in omega-3 PUFA prevented this rod dysfunction.[5] That's one reason why eating plenty of oily fish is a leading line of defence for people with diabetes.

Make sure you eat enough fish

Omega-3 PUFAs – specifically docosahexaenoic acid (DHA) and eicosapentaenoic acid (EPA) – seem to be responsible for much of oily fish's benefit. We can make omega-3 fatty acids from another fat, alpha-linolenic acid, found in green leafy vegetables, nuts, seeds and their oils. But it's a slow process. So, it's a good idea to boost levels by eating fish and seafood high in omega-3 fatty acids, such as tuna, salmon, herring, pilchard, mackerel, rainbow trout, dogfish, shrimp and crab. It's better to eat fresh fish. If you're eating canned fish, check the label to make sure processing has not depleted the omega-3 oils. It's also worth trying to check that the fish comes from sustainable stocks at <www.fishonline.org>.

The BDA advises that adults and children over 12 years should eat two portions of fish per week (a portion is about 140 g after cooking). One of these meals should be an oily fish. The BDA estimates that this will provide the equivalent of about 450 mg EPA/DHA per day. NICE advises that people who have experienced a heart attack should eat at least 7 g of omega-3 fatty acids per week from two to four portions of oily fish.

If at first you don't like the taste, don't give up without trying a few recipes. There's plenty of choice on the internet and in cookery books. For an island nation, our tastes in fish are remarkably conservative. However, avoid frying fish. Poach, grill or bake instead. And don't cover fish in breadcrumbs or batter, which can soak up fat. But if you really can't stomach the taste of oily fish you could try a supplement – provided you speak to your doctor first. Omega-3 supplements may increase blood sugar levels.

Oils, vitamin E and free radicals

If you a leave a slice of apple exposed to the air, it soon turns brown. A group of tissue-damaging chemicals called free radicals causes the colour change. Free radicals are a by-product of the normal chemical reactions that keep us alive. Our immune system uses free radicals to help destroy invading bacteria. Unfortunately, pollution, cigarette smoke, pesticides and even sunlight can generate free radicals that attack healthy cells. Excessive levels of free radicals seem to increase the risk of developing several serious conditions, including heart disease, cancer, stroke, Alzheimer's disease and rheumatoid arthritis. Levels of free radicals rise in diabetes, which may contribute to some of the potentially devastating complications.

Several lines of natural defence protect our delicate cells from free radicals: mostly members of a group of chemicals called antioxidants. Furthermore, several vitamins, minerals and other antioxidants in our diets mop up tissue-damaging free radicals, including:

- vitamins A, C, E and selenium;
- lutein, found in, for example, green leafy vegetables such as spinach and kale;
- lycopene, the red pigment in tomatoes and some other fruits.

Oils are a natural source of vitamin E, which is an important anti-oxidant. Unfortunately, processing removes vitamin E from some oils. Because they have fewer defences against attack from free radicals, processed oils are very susceptible to becoming rancid. So, ideally, obtain your fats from relatively unprocessed 'cold-pressed' vegetable oils, and natural sources such as seeds, nuts and oily fish. Cold-pressed oils should last longer and help bolster your antioxidant intake.

Vegetables, fruit and fibre

Our ancestors picked plants, fished and hunted. They ate vegetables, legumes, fruits and whole grains, which were usually fresh, often raw. This traditional diet is low GI, high in fibre and rich in vitamins and other micronutrients.[2] It's certainly a long way from processed ready meals and takeaway food. Many processed foods are loaded with sugar, salt and chemical additives such as preservatives, colourings and flavourings. Even white flour, bread and pasta are highly refined, which strips out many vitamins and nutrients.

As they lack key nutrients, processed foods can undermine your attempts at healthy eating. So, to eat a healthy diet you should cut down drastically on the processed foods in your diet, which can raise blood glucose levels.

Boost your fibre intake

Dietary fibre (roughage) is the part of plants that humans can't digest, such as the leaf webbing in green vegetables, the skins of sweetcorn and beans, and the husks of wheat and corn. There are two main types of fibre:

- Insoluble fibre remains largely intact as it moves through your digestive system, but eases defecation.
- Soluble fibre dissolves in water in the gut, forming a gel that soaks up fats. So a meal rich in soluble fibre means that you absorb less fat from a meal, which brings your blood cholesterol levels down. Soluble fibre also releases sugar slowly, producing steadier blood glucose concentrations after you eat.

Yet many of us don't eat sufficient fibre. Dieticians recommend that healthy adults should eat at least 18 g of fibre a day. European guidelines for diabetes suggest eating around 20 g of fibre for every 1,000 calories in your diet.[2] Currently, the average UK adult eats between 12 g and 14 g of fibre a day. So boost your consumption of:

- oats and oat bran
- fruit and vegetables
- nuts and seeds
- pulses – such as peas, soya, lentils and chickpeas
- wholemeal (wholegrain) breads and cereals (including wheat, oats, rye, barley and corn).

Fibre while you diet

Despite the popularity of high-protein, low-carbohydrate diets you should ensure you eat enough fibre, even while you are trying to lose weight. A high-fibre diet slowly releases carbohydrate. So you feel full for longer, reducing the risk that you will snack between meals. A low-carbohydrate diet makes it easier to not eat enough wholemeal foods, fruit and vegetables. As a result, you're less likely to consume sufficient fibre, vitamins and minerals.

Some people feel more thirsty when they eat a high-fibre diet. So try to drink about eight glasses of water a day. And don't mistake thirst for hunger.

Whole grains

Whole grains are an especially good source of fibre. Grains – the seeds of cereals, such as wheat, rye, barley, oats and rice – have three parts:

- Bran is the outer layer that is rich in fibre and packed with nutrients. It covers the germ and endosperm.
- The germ develops into a new plant and so is packed with nutrients. Wheat germ, for example, contains high levels of vitamin E, vitamin B_9 (folate/folic acid), zinc, magnesium and other valuable vitamins and minerals. In particular, a high intake of magnesium seems to reduce the risk of developing diabetes (page 110).[6]
- The central area (endosperm) is high in starch. The endosperm provides the energy the germ needs to develop into a new plant.

Food manufacturers refine grain by removing the bran and germ, and keeping the white endosperm. This removes most of the nutritional value. Indeed, wholegrain cereals contain up to 75 per cent more nutrients than refined cereals. Whole grains are rich in fibre and mop up tissue-damaging free radicals. Indeed, overwhelming evidence suggests that dietary fibre and whole grains protect against and help manage diabetes and related conditions, notably metabolic syndrome (page 25), obesity, hypertension, dyslipidaemia and cardiovascular disease.[6] Indeed, the BDA notes that regularly eating whole grains as part of a low-fat diet and a healthy lifestyle cuts the risk of heart disease by up to 30 per cent.

Whole grains seem to reduce the likelihood of developing diabetes by a similar amount to heart disease. For example, men who ate, on average, 10.2 g of cereal fibre a day were 30 per cent less likely to develop T2DM than those who ate just 2.5 g a day. In another study, women who consumed an average of 7.5 g of cereal fibre a day were 28 per cent less likely to develop diabetes than women who ate 2 g a day.[6]

Whole grains even help you control your weight by slowly releasing sugar into your blood. This, along with their high fibre content, means that you feel fuller for longer. You're less likely to snack because you feel hungry during the morning after a breakfast of porridge and wholegrain bread than one of refined cereals and white toast. The slow release may also mean you're less likely to snack to prevent your blood glucose levels falling towards the 'hypo zone'.

Despite these benefits, 95 per cent of adults in the UK don't eat enough whole grains. Nearly one-third don't eat any. The BDA suggests that you should aim to get at least half your starchy carbohydrates from whole grains, which means around two to three servings a day. Try eating more foods with 'whole' in front of the grain's name, such as wholewheat pasta and whole oats.

You should also try to consume a variety of whole grains, including oats, barley (generally available as pearl barley), corn, buckwheat, brown rice, maize and mixed grains. If you can't tolerate the gluten in wheat, try brown rice, millet, buckwheat, maize and corn, which are all gluten free. Here are some further tips for eating whole grains:

- Try to eat a bowl of porridge or muesli for breakfast every day, or toast made from stoneground wholewheat bread.

- Use brown or basmati rice instead of white rice.
- Use wholewheat pasta instead of refined white pasta.
- Include whole grains, such as barley, in soups and stews.
- Use bulgur wheat in casseroles and stir-fries.
- Substitute half the refined white flour in pancakes, buns and other flour-based recipes for wholewheat or oat flour. One of the authors prefers pancakes made totally with stoneground wholegrain flour than white flour.
- Use rolled oats or crushed unsweetened wholegrain cereal instead of bread to coat chicken, fish, veal cutlets and so on.
- Use wholegrain flour or oatmeal when making baked treats. Wholegrain muffins are an excellent choice.

What are whole foods?

Try to eat plenty of whole foods, which have had nothing taken away (such as nutrients and fibre) and nothing added (e.g. colourings, flavourings and preservatives). In short, foods in their most natural form. However, read the ingredient list carefully. Some brown bread is white bread coloured with added brown sugar.

Five portions of fruit and vegetables

You should ensure you eat five portions of fruit and vegetables a day: a portion weighs about 80 g. However, fruits are packed with a sugar called fructose. So eating large amounts of fruit in a short time can drive your blood glucose levels up. Examples of a portion of fruit and vegetables include:

- one medium-sized fruit (banana, apple, pear, orange)
- one slice of a large fruit (melon, pineapple, mango)
- two smaller fruits (plums, satsumas, apricots, peaches)
- a dessert bowl full of salad
- three heaped tablespoons of pulses (chickpeas, lentils, beans)
- two to three tablespoons (a handful) of grapes or berries
- one tablespoon of dried fruit
- one glass (150 ml) of unsweetened fruit or vegetable juice or smoothie. If you drink two or more glasses of juice a day, it still only counts as one portion.

To get the most benefit, eat your fruit and vegetables as raw as possible. Cooking can reduce the nutrient content. So, cook your vegetables using the minimum of unsalted (or lightly salted) water for the shortest time. Lightly steaming and stir-frying are healthy alternatives. Scrub rather than peel: the skin can contain valuable nutrients.

Drinking smoothies is another great way to boost your intake of fruit and vegetables. Two whole portions of fruit in a homemade smoothie counts as two of your five portions. However, some commercially available smoothies contain extra sugar, honey, yoghurt or milk that can increase the calorie, fat and sugar content. So always check the label.

If you find your usual basket of fruit and vegetables rather dull, try some more exotic alternatives. Different fruits and vegetables also provide different nutrients. You can also try the following to boost your intake:

- Snack on oranges, bananas or grapes during the day. Take them with you to work. Some employers will provide a fruit bowl in the office.
- Dried apricots, peaches and pineapple slices store well. You could keep a bag in your drawer at work.
- Buy packets of baby carrots or celery sticks to snack on.
- Add crushed fresh pineapple to coleslaw and add mandarin oranges or grapes to a tossed salad.
- Try baked apples, pears or a fruit salad for dessert.
- Make a variety of green salads and try to eat one every day as a main meal or a side salad. You can also take a salad to work with you in a plastic box.
- Plan some meals around vegetables rather than around meat, such as stir-fries, curries and soups.
- Add chopped vegetables to a pasta sauce or lasagne.
- To thicken and flavour a soup, stew or gravy, use cooked and pureed vegetables such as potatoes.
- When preparing a barbecue, try grilled vegetable kebabs.

Finally, try to buy locally grown, seasonal vegetables whenever possible. Levels of some nutrients decline between the farm and the plate, such as the time taken to transport food. But you can easily grow a crop of lettuce in a growing bag. Trim the leaves rather than uproot the plant and the crop can last all spring and summer. Beans and tomatoes are also easy to grow, even for the least green-fingered of us or in the smallest gardens. And gardening is a great way to exercise.

Some other tips to get the most benefit from fruit and vegetables include:

- Freeze any fruit and vegetables you can't eat straight away.
- If you can't get any fresh vegetables, try frozen, dried and tinned. But check the label to ensure that they don't contain added salt and sugar. When buying tinned fruit, choose those in 100 per cent fruit juice rather than syrup.
- Don't buy vegetables that come with sauces that contain added salt, sugar or fats. Even if you add a small pinch of salt you will still probably add far less than that in a normal tin of vegetables.
- Don't soak prepared fruit or vegetables, which may dissolve some vitamins and minerals.

The organic debate

Whether organic vegetables contain higher levels of nutrients than conventionally farmed produce is scientifically contentious. A recent study evaluated 33 studies encompassing 826 comparisons of the levels of micronutrients, such as vitamins and minerals, in organic and conventional foods. Levels of micronutrients were higher in organic foods in just over half (56 per cent) of the comparisons. But the difference was not that great. On average, levels of micronutrients were approximately 6 per cent higher in organic vegetables and legumes compared with their conventionally grown counterparts.[7] However, both authors of this book are convinced that organically farmed products are, overall, healthier – not least because they avoid pesticides and chemical fertilizers. Again, whether modern pesticides and chemical fertilizers used according to the rigorous rules applying in the UK cause widespread health problems is controversial. On the other hand, why eat them when you don't need to? And even a 6 per cent difference in nutrients could be worth having. So, if you feel like trying organic, don't be put off by the fruits' and vegetables' sometimes less than perfect shape.

Seeds, nuts and legumes

Seeds, nuts and legumes are another excellent source of fibre and other nutrients. Sunflower, sesame, hemp, flax and pumpkin seeds can be:

- eaten as snacks;
- sprinkled onto porridge and other breakfast cereals, as well as over salads;
- added to vegetable or meat dishes and soups;
- used in baking.

For more flavour, you could lightly roast the seeds after coating with soy sauce. Cracked linseed and pumpkin seeds are highly nutritious and can help alleviate constipation. However, seeds are relatively high in calories; the plant uses the stored energy to fuel germination and growth. So eat seeds in moderation if you are trying to lose weight.

Not all the nuts we eat are, strictly, nuts. Brazil and cashew nuts are seeds, for example. Peanuts are legumes, more closely related to peas and lentils than chestnuts and hazel nuts. You can ponder such scientific quibbles while eating a handful of almonds, cashews, walnuts, Brazils and pecans a day as snacks, with cereal and in baking. Obviously, if you are allergic to nuts, avoid them at all costs.

Legumes are a cheap source of protein (page 104), which is vital to the body for growth and maintenance, and have relatively little effect of blood glucose levels. Moreover, legumes are high in fibre and help control levels of fats in the blood, reducing the risk of cardiovascular disease and stroke. Legumes include:

- baked beans (but ideally choose a sugar-free version)
- kidney beans
- chickpeas
- red and green lentils
- mung beans
- butter beans
- black beans
- split peas
- haricot beans.

Use beans to add flavour to stews, soups, salads and casseroles and eat one to three portions of legumes daily. One portion is three heaped tablespoons of beans or peas.

Another legume – the soya bean – is particularly rich in PUFAs, especially linoleic (omega-6) and alpha-linolenic acid (omega-3), and low in saturated fat. One portion of soya beans counts towards the recommended five portions of fruits and vegetables a day, is high in fibre and, unlike most other plant foods, contains all the essential amino acids. Think about including soya derivatives in your diet, including soya milk, tofu, tempeh and miso. Tofu, for example, is very versatile and is used in both savoury and sweet dishes.

Soya milk

Some people prefer soya or rice milk, which is rich in protein, especially if they are lactose intolerant (although 1 person in every 200 is allergic to soya). However, it would be a good idea to ask your dietician or doctor to check whether you are really lactose intolerant. Other conditions – including irritable bowel syndrome – can cause similar symptoms. If you dislike soya milk and are lactose intolerant, your dietician can help you make up the nutrients you'll miss by removing milk from your diet.

Salt

According to the BDA, the average UK adult eats around 8.6 g of salt a day – that's about 2 teaspoons. However, the recommended intake for adults is 6 g of salt a day.

High levels of salt (sodium chloride) in your blood can damage your cells, so your body retains fluid to dilute the high levels of salt. But retaining fluid drives blood pressure up. That means that a high intake of salt makes it more likely you'll develop hypertension, which can lead to stroke and heart disease. Not surprisingly, if you take medication to lower your blood pressure (antihypertensives) and continue to eat a lot of salt there is a good chance that the medication will not be as effective as it should be. Drinking excess alcohol, smoking, avoiding exercise and eating a poor diet can also undermine the effectiveness of antihypertensives.

You can tell that some snacks are salty. But many foods contain hidden salt, so your taste buds won't warn you. Food producers add salt as a preservative and flavour enhancer to processed and prepackaged foods. For example:

- Manufacturers may add surprisingly large amounts of salt to some soups, bread, biscuits and breakfast cereals.
- Fresh chicken and turkey may be 'flavour enhanced' with added salt.
- 'Self-basting' poultry may mean that the manufacturer has added sodium and fat.
- Stock cubes are often high in salt.

Indeed, salt already added to food accounts for three-quarters of our intake. To cut your salt intake:

- Avoid foods that are high in salt, such as smoked meat and fish.
- Use as little salt as you can during cooking.
- Banish the salt cellar from the table.
- Ask restaurants and takeaways for no salt.
- Use only a very small amount of sea salt or rock salt in baking and cooking.
- Look for low-salt brands of ketchup, pickled items, mustard, yeast extract and stock cubes.

So, check the label and try to stick to low-salt foods. The BDA advises choosing meals and sandwiches with less than 0.5 g sodium (1.25 g salt) per meal. For individual foods, such as soups and sauces, choose those with under 0.3 g sodium (0.75 g) per serving. Some labels list the sodium rather than salt content. Chemically, table salt is sodium chloride. To convert sodium to salt multiply by 2.5. So, 0.4 g of sodium is 1 g of salt. You can convert salt to sodium by dividing by 2.5. Table 10 shows the amount of salt and sodium in high-, medium- and low-salt foods.

You may think your meals taste bland when you first reduce your salt use, but you will soon adjust to the new flavours. Indeed, in the space of a few weeks you will probably wonder why you preferred your foods so salty.

Table 10 Salt levels in food

Level	Salt content (per 100 g)	Sodium content (per 100 g)
High	More than 1.5 g	More than 0.6 g
Medium	0.3 g to 1.5 g	0.1 to 0.6 g
Low	0.3 g or less	0.1 g or less

Protein

Eating sufficient protein enables our bodies to repair and regenerate our tissues. Among many other actions, specialized proteins also:

- speed up chemical reactions essential for life (enzymes);
- act as receptors (page 7) for hormones and other messengers;
- form a scaffold that supports the cell's shape;
- are essential for fighting infections (antibodies).

So, not surprisingly, not eating enough protein can cause weakness, low energy, low stamina, poor resistance to infection, depression and slow wound healing. As mentioned above, people with diabetes are already particularly prone to some infections, delayed wound healing and depression. So a low-protein diet could make matters even worse.

However, while eating sufficient protein is essential for good health, it's important to get the balance right. For example:

- A high intake of protein seems to increase the risk of colon cancer. So, the government recommends that adults should avoid a protein intake that is more than twice the recommended level.
- The National Osteoporosis Society points out that a diet high in protein increases the acidity of the blood and other fluids in the body (proteins are made from long chains of amino acids). This may draw minerals, including calcium, from the skeleton.
- People who eat large amounts of red meat may be between 24 and 36 per cent more likely to develop diabetes. And it's the protein, rather than just the saturated fat, that's to blame.[6]
- As mentioned in Chapter 1, the body can convert certain amino acids to glucose. So, a meal that's very high in protein and low in carbohydrate can still result in high levels of blood glucose several hours after eating.[8]

Unless you eat very large amounts, protein-rich foods have little impact on blood glucose levels. However, some protein-rich foods include carbohydrate added by the manufacturer. Sausages may include cereals. Fish fingers and chicken nuggets are coated in breadcrumbs, while meat pies, sausage rolls and quiches obviously include pastry.

How much is enough?

The BDA suggests that the general sedentary population should eat 0.80–1.0 g of protein per kg bodyweight each day. Endurance athletes (1.2–1.4 g per kg body weight) and strength athletes (1.2–1.7 g per kg body weight) need slightly more. In general, protein should account for just less than one-third of what is on your plate at each meal.

Provided you don't have kidney damage, European guidelines for diabetes suggest that protein should account for between 10 and 20 per cent of your daily energy intake. However, your diabetes team may recommend reducing your intake to about 0.8 g of protein for each kg of body weight if you have established nephropathy.[9] But *if you have kidney damage don't change your protein intake without speaking to a dietician first.*

Sources of protein

Protein sources include chicken, turkey, fish, beans and legumes. However, animal protein can be loaded with saturated fat. So try to eat fresh, lean cuts of meat (see below for some suggestions). Ideally, you should eat a serving of meat no larger or thicker than the palm of your hand on no more than two occasions a week. Try to avoid poultry coated in breadcrumbs or batter, which will boost blood glucose levels. And ideally eat free-range or organically produced meat to avoid pesticides, antibiotics and hormones used in animal husbandry. The rest of your protein intake should come from other sources, such as fish, poultry, soya products, organic live yoghurt, nuts, seeds and legumes.

Poultry, such as chicken and turkey, contains less fat than red meat. So eat chicken or turkey once or twice a week. Dairy foods are rich in protein. However, you should always read the label and try to select low-fat products and choose yoghurt with no added sugar. You could also try low-fat cheeses (including spreads) in moderation. Here are some other suggestions for buying, cooking and eating meat:

- Choose the leanest cuts of meat you can find:
  - Beef : top loin, top sirloin and shoulder beef
  - Pork: pork loin, tenderloin and ham
  - Lamb: the shank half of the leg
  - Poultry: boneless chicken breasts and turkey cutlets.

- Trim any visible fat before cooking. You can ask a butcher to do this.
- Grill, roast, poach or boil meat instead of frying.
- If you must fry meat, avoid coating in breadcrumbs, which soaks up fat.
- Choose extra-lean minced meat. Ideally, avoid mince altogether.
- Drain any fat released from cooking.
- If you can't resist the occasional burger or sausage, check the label and choose processed meats with less saturated fat.

Following a healthy, balanced diet and using your medicines as suggested by your diabetes team should help you control your blood glucose level and reduce your risk of developing long-term complications. However, some people feel that they need additional support from supplements, which we'll look at in the next chapter.

10

Using supplements safely

In theory, you should have no need for vitamin and mineral supplements if you eat a healthy balanced diet as recommended in this book. Nevertheless, some people still regard a vitamin supplement as an insurance policy. Others feel that they would like to try a herbal treatment to keep their glucose levels down or tackle a diabetic complication.

For most people without diabetes, vitamin and most herbal supplements don't do any harm. However, people with diabetes need to be careful, especially those using insulin or some other antidiabetic drugs. Some supplements interact with diabetes medications. Manganese and vanadium, for example, both augment insulin's action[1] and could trigger a hypo.

If you read that a supplement helps a particular diabetes-related problem there's often an alternative dietary source. If you want to try a supplement you *must* check with your diabetes care team first. Even if you're using diet alone to manage your T2DM or you are still in prediabetes you will need to check the supplement won't interact with any other medications that you're taking for other conditions, such as heart disease, raised blood pressure, arthritis and so on. For example, St John's wort (used for depression) can interact with the contraceptive pill. *Everyone taking a medicine for any disease, including insulin or any drug for T2DM, MUST speak to a doctor or diabetes nurse before embarking on a course of supplements.*

A common misconception

There's a common misconception that because supplements are natural they are safe. But high doses of vitamins can be dangerous, even if you don't have diabetes. In 1596, Dutch sailors exploring the Arctic island of Novaya Zemlya fell dangerously ill after eating polar bear liver. Three sailors lost their skin 'from head to foot'. Many subsequent expeditions fell victim to the same malady. We now know that polar bear livers contain very high levels of vitamin A. You're unlikely to consume enough vitamin A to experience the same reaction, but it remains a sobering reminder that while sufficient vitamins and minerals are essential for health, excessive levels can be dangerous. Not all products include the detailed information you need to take the supplement safely. So talk to your doctor or nurse before trying a supplement or indeed any complementary treatment.

In general, Diabetes UK does not recommend that people with diabetes should take a supplement, with the exception of folic acid during pregnancy. But if you're taking insulin or a drug for diabetes and you're convinced that a supplement will help – and your doctor or nurse agrees – you must keep an even closer eye on your blood glucose levels.

Folic acid

Every woman who is, or is planning to become, pregnant should take a folic acid supplement. The body converts the folic acid to folate (also called vitamin B_9) and uses it in numerous ways, including making DNA. So it's essential to make new cells. Unfortunately, you don't store much folate. As a result you need a regular fresh supply of folic acid to keep healthy, from vegetables such as spinach, sprouts, broccoli, green beans and potatoes and fortified bread and breakfast cereals.

Taking folic acid supplements in early pregnancy reduces the risk of neural tube defects such as spina bifida, where the backbone and spinal canal do not close properly before birth. Diabetes seems to increase the risk of neural tube defects.[2] So, women with diabetes who are, or are planning to become, pregnant should take a higher dose (5 mg) of folic acid than those without diabetes during the first 12 weeks of pregnancy. Talk to your midwife or diabetes team as soon as you know you want to have a baby or discover that you're pregnant.

Alpha-lipoic acid

Cells produce a chemical called alpha-lipoic acid to help generate energy. Alpha-lipoic acid, also known as thioctic acid, mops up free radicals and helps cells recycle other antioxidants that include vitamins C and E. Furthermore, alpha-lipoic acid improves blood flow to nerves and enhances nerve conduction.[3,4] In diabetes, alpha-lipoic acid seems to:

- prevent destruction of beta cells;
- enhance glucose uptake by cells;
- slow the development of diabetic complications, including neuropathy.

Indeed, doctors in Germany can prescribe alpha-lipoic acid to treat diabetic neuropathy. In the UK, you should be able to buy alpha-lipoic acid from health food shops. But high doses of alpha-lipoic acid can cause headache, rash, stomach upsets and trigger hypoglycaemia.[3,4] So, as always, if you're taking any medicine for diabetes don't take alpha-lipoic acid without speaking to a health care professional first.

Calcium

Most of the calcium in your body (about 1 kg in a 70 kg person) helps build strong bones and teeth. Around 1 per cent has other critical roles, such as ensuring efficient nerve transmission, controlling hormone secretion and allowing muscle contraction.

Consuming enough calcium helps protect against brittle bone disease (osteoporosis). The National Osteoporosis Society suggests that adults need 700 mg of calcium a day. Breastfeeding mothers and people with osteoporosis may need more: in the latter case between 1,200 and 1,500 mg of calcium a day. To put this in context:

- Half a pint (280 ml) of calcium-enriched soya milk contains 370 mg of calcium.
- Half a pint of skimmed milk contains 355 mg of calcium.
- Two tinned pilchards contain 275 mg.
- A 150 g pot of yoghurt contains 225 mg.
- 30 g of cheddar cheese contains 220 mg.
- Two large slices of white or brown bread contain 130 mg.
- Two large slices of wholemeal bread contain 75 mg.

But the amount of calcium in foods can vary from product to product. So read the label. If you feel you can't get enough calcium from your diet you could consider taking a supplement. However, one study found that over an average of 4 years people taking a calcium supplement were 27 per cent more likely to experience a heart attack. Overall, treating 1,000 people with calcium for 5 years would cause 14 extra heart attacks, 10 more strokes and a further 13 deaths, while preventing 26 fractures.[5] So again, check with your doctor first, especially if you have a history of heart disease.

Chromium

Chromium boosts the action of insulin and helps the body use protein, fat and carbohydrate effectively. In some animal studies, chromium supplements prevented the development of diabetes. For example, the soil in some parts of China contains little chromium. So, people living in these regions are severely deficient in this vital mineral. In such instances, chromium supplementation reverses some cases of diabetes.[6] Whole grains, meat, egg yolk, mushrooms and meat are rich in chromium.

Magnesium

Several studies suggest that magnesium reduces diabetes risk. Overall, an intake of approximately 400 mg of magnesium a day seems to reduces diabetes risk by around 33 per cent compared with an intake of about 250 mg a day.[6] You could boost your consumption by eating more whole grains, legumes, nuts and beans, all of which are rich in this essential mineral.

Vanadium

Large doses (100–125 mg/day) of vanadium improve cells' sensitivity to insulin in humans. But at these doses, vanadium tends to cause side effects such as abdominal discomfort, diarrhoea, nausea, flatulence, loss of energy and even a green tongue. Future studies need to investigate whether vanadium is safe and effective in preventing diabetes.[6]

Vitamin B$_{12}$ (cyanocobalamin)

Vitamin B$_{12}$ is essential:

- for formation of red blood cells;
- to produce DNA;
- to make sure your nerves work properly;
- and to help the body use fat and protein effectively.

Only animal products, such as oily fish, seafood, meat, eggs, milk and poultry naturally contain vitamin B$_{12}$. However, some breakfast cereals are fortified with vitamin B$_{12}$, which is good news for vegetarians and vegans.

Some studies suggest that vitamin B$_{12}$ supplements improve diabetic neuropathy (see page 49), reducing pain and paraesthesia (sensations such as tingling, burning, pricking, and pins and needles). Vitamin B$_{12}$ supplements may also alleviate the autonomic symptoms caused by nerve damage, which include constipation, diarrhoea, impotence, dry skin and poor awareness of hypoglycaemia. Further studies are needed to confirm the extent of the benefits.[7,8] Nevertheless, if you've developed neuropathy it might be worth speaking to your diabetes team about taking a vitamin B$_{12}$ supplement.

Vitamin C (ascorbic acid)

Vitamin C is one of the body's most important defences against tissue-damaging free radicals (page 94). Levels of free radicals rise in diabetes, which may contribute to some complications. Vitamin C may also reduce formation of a sugar called sorbitol that's linked to retinopathy, neuropathy and kidney damage.

Unfortunately, people with diabetes don't seem to have enough of this important antioxidant. In one study, 56 per cent of people with diabetes showed low levels of vitamin C in their blood.[9] Other studies suggest that, on average, people with diabetes have vitamin C levels at least 30 per cent lower than healthy people. While vitamin C supplements don't seem to markedly change blood glucose levels, sorbitol levels decline and the capillaries may become less fragile.[10] Raw cabbage, carrots, lettuce, onions, celery, tomatoes, oranges, lemons, limes, grapefruits and all other citrus fruits are good sources of vitamin C.

Herbal supplements

In 1960, archaeologists discovered a Neanderthal skeleton buried in caves in Shanidar, Iraq. Several plants used by modern herbalists, including cornflower, yarrow and groundsel, surrounded the remains. Almost certainly, the plants weren't there by accident. They probably formed part of the Neanderthals' pharmacy.

Even today, herbs remain the main source of medicines for much of humanity and are popular even in countries able to afford modern medicines. Indeed, many medicines prescribed by your doctor – even for serious diseases such as diabetes and cancer – and available from pharmacists trace their origins to herbs.

For example, in 1962, a botanist called Arthur Barclay peeled some bark from a Pacific yew tree (*Taxus brevifolia*) growing in the Gifford Pinchot National Forest in north-eastern USA. Two years later, researchers recognized that an extract from the bark inhibited the growth of cancer cells.[11] They isolated a drug called paclitaxel from the bark. Today oncologists use paclitaxel to treat various malignancies, including lung, breast and ovarian cancer. A plaque commemorates where Barclay took his sample.[11]

Paclitaxel isn't an isolated example. In 1763, an English cleric, Edward Stone, found that willow bark alleviated ague, a fever linked to malaria, which was rife in England at the time. Aspirin is a chemically modified, less toxic version of the active ingredient in willow bark. As a final example, metformin – one of the most important diabetes drugs (page 59) – is a chemical modification of substances in a plant known as goat's rue or French lilac (*Galega officinalis*). Medieval healers used *G. officinalis* to relieve the urinary problems accompanying diabetes.

Not surprisingly, herbs may occasionally interact with medicines used to treat diabetes and may undermine control of your blood glucose. Indeed, fenugreek (*Trigonella foenum-graecum*) can lower blood glucose levels to a similar extent as insulin.[1] Such potent glucose-lowering actions could trigger a hypo if you're on insulin or some other antidiabetic drugs.

So, it is worth repeating the earlier warning: if you're using diet alone to treat T2DM or you are still in prediabetes some of these herbal supplements may help control your blood glucose levels, although you still need to check the supplement won't interact with any medicines that you're taking for other conditions. *Everyone taking a medicine for any disease, including those with T1DM and T2DM, MUST speak to a doctor or diabetes nurse before taking a herbal treatment – even if you can buy it from a health shop.*

You should also make sure you buy any herbs from a reputable source. In the 1990s, testing revealed that some natural treatments for diabetes were laced with glucose-lowering drugs, including glibenclamide.[12] *Indeed, if you have prediabetes or are trying to control T2DM with lifestyle changes alone is best to be treated by a qualified medical herbalist and make sure that they know you have prediabetes, diabetes and any other medical conditions.* However, the following herbs may help some people control their blood glucose levels and manage some diabetic complications.

Bitter melon

Bitter melon (*Momordica charantia*; also called bitter gourd or balsam pear) is a traditional treatment for diabetes that is still widely used across Asia, South America, India and East Africa. Numerous experimental studies performed since the 1950s show that bitter melon lowers blood glucose levels and tackles diabetes. Indeed, in some studies bitter melon reduced blood glucose as much as tolbutamide, chlorpropamide and glibenclamide (see Chapter 5).[13]

Bitter melon seems to act in several ways to help cells use glucose more efficiently and reduce insulin resistance. In one study of people with T2DM, bitter melon reduced glucose levels by, on average, about one-fifth (18 per cent). Furthermore, around 9 in 10 patients benefited (86 per cent). Other clinical studies confirm that bitter melon lowers glucose levels in humans. Gastrointestinal upset is a possible side effect and children occasionally developed diabetic coma after drinking bitter melon tea.[13] Further investigations are needed to fully define bitter melon's benefits.

Evening primrose oil

Oil from the seeds of the evening primrose (*Oenothera biennis*) are high in omega-3 and omega-6 polyunsaturated fatty acids (see page 92), such as gamma-linolenic acid and linoleic acid. These fatty acids are essential components of the myelin sheath that surrounds each nerve and for the nerve cells' membrane. Indeed, some studies involving people with diabetic neuropathy found that evening primrose oil might improve nerve function and alleviate symp-toms. However, once again, more studies are needed before doctors can routinely suggest the treatment.[3] But if you want to try evening primrose oil speak to your doctor or diabetes nurse specialist.

Fenugreek

Fenugreek seems to stimulate insulin secretion from the pancreas and reduce insulin resistance. Indeed, in some studies, fenugreek lowered blood glucose to a similar extent as insulin. Fenugreek seeds contain about 30 per cent soluble fibre and 20 per cent insol-uble fibre. So fenugreek seeds also slow the rate at which you absorb glucose from a meal, which probably contributes to their benefits. In addition, fenugreek reduces levels of triglycerides, cholesterol and LDL-cholesterol in your blood.[1]

Ginseng

Ginseng (*Panax ginseng* and *Panax quinquefolius*) seems to boost the immune system, reduce inflammation and mop up tissue-damaging free radicals. So, ginseng seems to reduce the risk of cardiovascular disease and infections – and is also one of the best studied antidiabetic herbs.[14]

Ginseng seems to improve the transfer of glucose into energy and protects insulin-producing beta cells in the pancreas (page 4) from destruction. In one study using obese diabetic mice, ginseng reduced the peak in glucose in the 2 hours after eating by 46 per cent. Ginseng also normalized insulin levels and reduced choles-terol levels and weight. In studies of people with T2DM ginseng, among other benefits, blunted the surge in blood glucose levels after a meal, reduced HbA_{1c} (see page 37) and fasting glucose levels, and increased levels of physical activity.[14]

Prickly pear

Several small studies suggest that the prickly pear (*Opuntia humifusa*) may lower blood glucose levels. For example, in an experiment using diabetic rats, an extract of the stem of prickly pear reduced levels of blood glucose, triglycerides, cholesterol and LDL-cholesterol, while boosting levels of the healthy HDL-cholesterol (page 27).[15] If this high-fibre fruit is not available in your local greengrocer, you could drink prickly pear as a powder or juice from a health food shop.

Benefits and limitations

Numerous other herbs and supplements may improve diabetes, according to scientific studies, medical traditions or both. But the examples above give you a flavour of the benefits and limitations – usually that supplements can cause side effects and that more studies are needed.

Certainly, few complementary therapies undergo the same rigorous scrutiny as modern medicines. But clinical studies are expensive and pharmaceutical companies fund most trials. So this lack of studies isn't that surprising. It's worth remembering that no evidence of effectiveness isn't necessarily the same as evidence of no effect. Nevertheless, if you fail to see any benefits after 3 months you should stop using the supplement. And before you embark on a course of herbal supplements, speak to your GP or diabetes care team. Ideally, don't treat yourself, but see a qualified medical herbalist – and make sure they know you have diabetes.

11

Putting it all together

Managing diabetes can be a pain, literally, if you inject insulin or measure blood glucose levels. And juggling diabetes alongside your other commitments often proves difficult. Yet, despite the need to stick to a routine, despite the need to take medicines regularly, despite the need to follow a healthy, balanced diet, you're not a slave to your diabetes. Some people worry enormously if they are as little as 2 minutes late taking their diabetes medication, or if they are slightly behind in checking their blood glucose levels. But a few minutes rarely matters.

Where diet is concerned, it's not worth getting into a panic because you could not resist tucking into that delicious sweet pudding. For a very small number of people with diabetes, rigid dietary control is essential. But most people with diabetes can be flexible on occasion. However, you may need to adjust your dose of insulin to redress the balance. If you have T2DM you need to make sure that the pudding isn't the first step on a slippery slope back to your old dietary habits.

So what conclusions can we draw from our look at healthy eating in diabetes? Following the top ten healthy diet tips (see box) will help you keep your blood glucose levels under control and reduce the risk of complications. However, as you change your diet – even for the better – you'll need to keep an eye on your blood glucose level. Assuming, of course, you're not changing your lifestyle to tackle prediabetes or treat early T2DM. Essentially, we suggest you test your blood glucose levels as suggested by your diabetes care team. Then, tailor your treatment based on your blood glucose levels. Your diabetes team can help you if you have any concerns.

A healthy, balanced diet as outlined in this book should help you lose any excess weight and stay at a healthy BMI (page 18). If you can eat healthily, have portions of the recommended size and be more active, you will lose weight. This may mean you need

The ten golden rules for a diabetic diet

1 Eat three meals a day containing a variety of foods; remember that you should never skip breakfast.
3 Include starchy carbohydrates in each meal.
3 Eat a fairly low-fat diet, with little saturated fat.
4 Eat plenty of grains and legumes (e.g. beans and lentils).
5 Eat at least two portions of oily fish each week.
6 Cut down on sugary foods and use less table sugar.
7 Drink alcohol in moderation – and never exceed the recommendation made by your diabetes team.
8 Cut down on salt.
9 Cut down on processed foods – eat more whole grains.
10 Eat five portions of fruit and vegetables a day.

Expanded from Diabetes UK

less medication to control your blood sugar levels. It's important that you speak to your doctor or diabetes care team about how to safely reduce your dose. But even if the drugs remain the same, the healthy balanced diet will help you reduce the risk that you'll develop the serious complications often linked to diabetes.

Some food choices

A healthy, balanced diet does not have to be boring. Table 11 shows that you can eat a wide range of foods. You can obviously mix and match the columns; many of the lunch suggestions can work equally well as an evening meal, especially if you have to work and can't cook in the office. And these are just suggestions. Look in your cookery books – they don't need to cater especially for people with diabetes. Just make sure the recipes focus on healthy eating and, ideally, give you an idea of the nutrient content. Then choose the foods that appeal to you based around the principles that we have outlined in the book.

Table 11 Suggested menus for healthy eating for people with diabetes

Breakfast	Snack	Lunch	Snack	Evening meal
Oat porridge with a sprinkling of cracked linseed	One banana or two satsumas	Baked potato with sugar-free baked beans and salad; low-fat blueberry muffin	Cereal bar*	Chicken or vegetable curry with wholegrain or basmati rice; Greek yoghurt
Muesli with sliced fruit and skimmed milk	Low-fat bio-yoghurt	Boiled egg, two slices of wholegrain bread and a scraping of butter	Two kiwi fruits	Salad with fresh prawns and low-fat dip; slice of fruit cake*
All-Bran with sliced fruit and skimmed milk	Popcorn	Falafel in pitta bread	Low-fat muffin	Chicken, vegetable or tofu stir-fry with wholegrain noodles; fruit salad
Two poached eggs on toasted wholemeal bread	Fruit loaf*	Mixed grain bread	A small handful of sesame seeds or raw slices of carrot	Wholemeal pasta with tomato and coriander sauce; blackberry and apple crumble
Two crumpets with low-fat spread	Small handful of nuts (unsalted)	Baked salmon with lemon and olive oil dressing, potato, broccoli and peas	Small handful of dried chopped pineapple	Lentil and tomato soup; pears cooked in red wine

Breakfast	Snack	Lunch	Snack	Evening meal
Grilled kippers and two rye biscuits	Two slices of wholemeal toast with a little butter and low-sugar marmalade	Soup with pearl barley; low-fat yoghurt	Handful of mixed nuts	Grilled herring with fresh salad; tinned peaches in fruit juice
Porridge made with skimmed milk and topped with dried fruits	Carrot sticks	Lamb casserole with plenty of vegetables; small handful of olives	Small handful of dried apricots	Low-fat burger in a wholegrain bap with side salad; watermelon
Tomato and mushroom omelette	Two oat biscuits	Lettuce, tomato and cucumber sandwich on wholemeal bread	Banana	Chicken or turkey salad with olive oil and vinegar dressing; sliced banana with Greek yoghurt
Boiled egg with wholemeal bread and low-fat spread	One slice fruit malt loaf*	Bean risotto; baked egg custard	Apple	Carrot and coriander soup; low-fat ice cream
One wholemeal blueberry muffin*	Slice of pumpernickel bread with a scraping of butter	Two poached eggs with grilled bacon, tomato and mushrooms	Chopped raw vegetables with low-fat dip	Tomato soup; low-fat ice cream with strawberries

*Eat limited amounts if you're trying to lose weight.

Eat regularly

If you have diabetes, especially T1DM or if you take drugs for T2DM, you should not skip meals and ideally space your breakfast, lunch and evening meal evenly over the day. Regular meals help everyone avoid hunger pangs, control their appetite and maintain stable blood glucose levels. On the other hand, eating irregular large meals can cause a dramatic rise in blood glucose levels.[1] And remember that poor coordination between eating and insulin dosing causes many hypos.

You'll need to find the pattern of meals that's right for you. Some people eat three meals a day. Others need some snacks between meals to ensure they don't move towards the 'hypo zone'. Table 11 has some healthy snack suggestions. If possible, it's better to eat a more substantial lunch than evening meal as the body has longer to digest the food. You will also, if necessary, be able to keep a closer eye on your blood glucose and watch for any symptoms of hyperglycaemia or hypos. Wait for at least 3 hours after eating your evening meal before going to bed – a full stomach can disturb sleep. If you need to you can eat a light snack in the meantime.

You are what you eat

The basic idea of controlling diabetes is relatively simple: keep levels of blood glucose low enough to avoid immediate and long-term complications, and tackle the other risk factors. But, in practice, controlling diabetes often proves difficult and needs a multipronged approach. Nevertheless, eating a healthy balanced diet is likely to remain the keystone of management for people with diabetes.

We have come a long way since Frederick Madison Allen suggested cutting carbohydrate consumption to starvation levels. We now know that diet is rarely the sole answer, although combined with other lifestyle changes a healthy, balanced choice of foods often slows the progression or, in some cases, even reverses the progression of early T2DM. A healthy, balanced diet underpins other elements in the care of people with diabetes – even in T1DM and advanced T2DM. After all, you are what you eat.

Useful addresses

Action on Smoking and Health (ASH)
First Floor
144–145 Shoreditch High Street
London E1 6JE
Tel.: 020 7739 5902
Website: www.ash.org.uk

Alcohol Concern
Suite B5, West Wing
New City Cloisters
196 Old Street
London EC1V 9FR
Tel.: 020 7566 9800
Website: www.alcoholconcern.org.uk

American Diabetes Association
ATTN: Center for Information
1701 North Beauregard Street
Alexandria
VA 22311
USA
Tel.: 1-800-DIABETES (800-343-2383)
Website: www.diabetes.org

British Association for Counselling and Psychotherapy
BACP House
15 St John's Business Park
Lutterworth LE17 4HB
Tel.: 01455 883300
Website: www.bacp.co.uk

British Association of Medical Hypnosis
45 Hyde Park Square
London W2 2JT
Website: www.bamh.org.uk

British Chiropody and Podiatry Association
New Hall
149 Bath Road
Maidenhead
Berkshire SL6 4LA
Tel.: 01628 632440
Website: www.bcha-uk.org

British Dietetic Association
Fifth Floor, Charles House
148/9 Great Charles Street Queensway
Birmingham B3 3HT
Tel.: 0121 200 8080
Website: www.bda.uk.com

British Heart Foundation
Greater London House
180 Hampstead Road
London NW1 7AW
Helpline: 0300 330 3311 (Monday to Friday, 9 a.m. to 5 p.m.)
Website: www.bhf.org.uk
For BHF's statistics on heart disease, go to <www.bhf.org.uk/research/
statistics.aspx>

Diabetes Research and Wellness Foundation
101–102 Northney Marina
Hayling Island
Hampshire PO11 0NH
Tel.: 023 92 637808
Website: www.drwf.org.uk

Diabetes UK
Macleod House
10 Parkway
London NW1 7AA
Tel.: 020 7424 1000; CareLine 0845 1202960
Website: www.diabetes.org.uk

Health Professions Council
Park House
184 Kennington Park Road
London SE11 4BU
Tel.: 0845 300 6184 (8 a.m. to 6 p.m., weekdays)
Website: www.hpc-uk.org

**Institute for Complementary and Natural Medicine (and British
Register of Complementary Practitioners)**
Can-Mezzanine
32–36 Loman Street
London SE1 0EH
Tel.: 020 7922 7980
Website: www.icnm.org.uk

Institute of Chiropodists and Podiatrists
27 Wright Street
Southport
Merseyside PR9 0TL
Tel.: 01704 546141
Website: www.iocp.org.uk

Insulin Dependent Diabetes Trust
PO Box 294
Northampton NN1 4XS
Tel.: 01604 622 837 (confidential helpline, 9 a.m. to 5 p.m., Monday to Friday)
Website: www.iddt.org

International Diabetes Federation
166 Chaussee de La Hulpe
B-1170 Brussels
Belgium
Tel.: +32-2-538 55 11
Website: www.idf.org

Juvenile Diabetes Research Foundation
19 Angel Gate
City Road
London EC1V 2PT
Tel.: 020 7713 2030
Website: www.jdrf.org.uk

Kidney Research UK
Nene Hall
Lynch Wood Park
Peterborough PE2 6FZ
Tel.: 0845 070 7601 (general); 0845 300 1499 (for specific information on kidney-health issues)
Website: www.kidneyresearchuk.org

National Health Service (advice on stopping smoking)
NHS Smoking Helpline: 0800 022 4 332
Website: www.smokefree.nhs.uk

National Kidney Federation
The Point
Coach Road
Shireoaks
Worksop
Nottinghamshire S81 8BW
Tel.: 01909 544999 (general); 0845 601 02 09 (patients' helpline, 9 a.m. to 5 p.m., Monday to Friday)
Website: www.kidney.org.uk

National Osteoporosis Society
Camerton
Bath BA2 0PJ
Helpline: 0845 450 0230 (9 a.m. to 5 p.m., Monday to Friday)
Website: www.nos.org.uk

Royal National Institute of Blind People
105 Judd Street
London WC1H 9NE
Tel.: 020 7388 1266 (general); 0303 123 9999 (helpline)
Website: www.rnib.org.uk

Society of Chiropodists and Podiatrists
1 Fellmonger's Path
Tower Bridge Road
London SE1 3LY
Tel.: 020 7234 8620
Website: www.feetforlife.org

Stroke Association
Stroke House
240 City Road
London EC1V 2PR
Tel.: 020 7566 0300 (general); 0303 303 3100 (helpline)
Website: www.stroke.org.uk

References

Introduction

1 Mazur A. Why were "starvation diets" promoted for diabetes in the pre-insulin period? *Nutrition Journal.* 2011; **10**: 23.
2 Cox C. Elizabeth Evans Hughes—surviving starvation therapy for diabetes. *Lancet.* 2011; **377**(9773): 1232–3.
3 Tattersall R. *Diabetes: The Biography.* Oxford: Oxford University Press; 2009.

1 The pancreas – controlling glucose levels

1 Tattersall R. *Diabetes: The Biography.* Oxford: Oxford University Press; 2009.
2 Sakula A. Paul Langerhans (1847–1888): a centenary tribute. *Journal of the Royal Society of Medicine.* 1988; **81**(7): 414–5.
3 Mazze RS, Strock ES, Bergenstal RM, Criego A, Cuddihy R, Langer O, et al. Detection and treatment of type 1 diabetes. In: *Staged Diabetes Management.* Wiley-Blackwell; 2011, p. 41–75.

2 Types of diabetes and their symptoms

1 Tattersall R. *Diabetes: The Biography.* Oxford: Oxford University Press; 2009.
2 Cox C. Elizabeth Evans Hughes—surviving starvation therapy for diabetes. *Lancet.* 2011; **377**(9773): 1232–3.
3 Matthews D, Beatty S, Dyson P, King L, Meston N, Pal A, et al. *Diabetes: The Facts.* Oxford: Oxford University Press; 2008.
4 Thanabalasingham G, Owen KR. Diagnosis and management of maturity onset diabetes of the young (MODY). *BMJ.* 2011; **343**: d6044.
5 Mazze RS, Strock ES, Bergenstal RM, Criego A, Cuddihy R, Langer O, et al. Detection and treatment of type 1 diabetes. In: *Staged Diabetes Management.* Wiley-Blackwell; 2011, p. 41–75.
6 Pitkaniemi J, Onkamo P, Tuomilehto J, Arjas E. Increasing incidence of type 1 diabetes—role for genes? *BMC Genetics.* 2004; **5**: 5.
7 Rosenfeld L. Insulin: discovery and controversy. *Clinical Chemistry.* 2002; **48**(12): 2270–88.

8 Mazze RS, Strock ES, Bergenstal RM, Criego A, Cuddihy R, Langer O, et al. Type 2 diabetes in adults. In: *Staged Diabetes Management*. Wiley-Blackwell; 2011, p. 77–137.

9 Glucose tolerance and cardiovascular mortality: comparison of fasting and 2-hour diagnostic criteria. *Archives of Internal Medicine*. 2001; **161**(3): 397–405.

10 Aroda VR, Ratner R. Approach to the patient with prediabetes. *Journal of Clinical Endocrinology and Metabolism*. 2008; **93**(9): 3259–65.

11 Choudhuri G, Lakshmi C, Goel A. Pancreatic diabetes. *Tropical Gastroenterology*. 2009; **30**: 71–5.

12 Suissa S, Kezouh A, Ernst P. Inhaled corticosteroids and the risks of diabetes onset and progression. *American Journal of Medicine*. 2010; **123**(11): 1001–6.

3 Risk factors for diabetes

1 Parkin DM, Boyd L. 4. Cancers attributable to dietary factors in the UK in 2010. *British Journal of Cancer*. 2011; **105**(S2): S19–23.

2 Tattersall R. *Diabetes: The Biography*. Oxford: Oxford University Press; 2009.

3 Yusuf S, Hawken S, Ounpuu S, Dans T, Avezum A, Lanas F, et al. Effect of potentially modifiable risk factors associated with myocardial infarction in 52 countries (the INTERHEART study): case-control study. *Lancet*. 2004; **364**(9438): 937–52.

4 Hodge AM, English DR, O'Dea K, Giles GG. Alcohol intake, consumption pattern and beverage type, and the risk of type 2 diabetes. *Diabetic Medicine*. 2006; **23**(6): 690–7.

5 Cullmann M, Hilding A, Östenson CG. Alcohol consumption and risk of pre-diabetes and type 2 diabetes development in a Swedish population. *Diabetic Medicine*. 2012; **29**(4): 441–52.

6 Kao WH, Puddey IB, Boland LL, Watson RL, Brancati FL. Alcohol consumption and the risk of type 2 diabetes mellitus: atherosclerosis risk in communities study. *American Journal of Epidemiology*. 2001; **154**(8): 748–57.

7 Matthews D, Beatty S, Dyson P, King L, Meston N, Pal A, et al. *Diabetes: The Facts*. Oxford: Oxford University Press; 2008.

4 Complications of poorly controlled diabetes

1 Baquer NZ, Kumar P, Taha A, Kale RK, Cowsik SM, McLean P. Metabolic and molecular action of *Trigonella foenum-graecum* (fenugreek) and trace metals in experimental diabetic tissues. *Journal of Biosciences*. 2011; **36**(2): 383–96.

2 Tattersall R. *Diabetes: The Biography*. Oxford: Oxford University Press; 2009.

3 Mazze RS, Strock ES, Bergenstal RM, Criego A, Cuddihy R, Langer O, et al. Detection and treatment of type 1 diabetes. In: *Staged Diabetes Management*. Wiley-Blackwell; 2011, p. 41–75.

4 The effect of intensive treatment of diabetes on the development and progression of long-term complications in insulin-dependent diabetes mellitus. *New England Journal of Medicine*. 1993; **329**(14): 977–86.

5 Stratton IM, Adler AI, Neil HA, Matthews DR, Manley SE, Cull CA, et al. Association of glycaemia with macrovascular and microvascular complications of type 2 diabetes (UKPDS 35): prospective observational study. *BMJ*. 2000; **321**(7258): 405–12.

6 Mazze RS, Strock ES, Bergenstal RM, Criego A, Cuddihy R, Langer O, et al. Type 2 diabetes in adults. In: *Staged Diabetes Management*. Wiley-Blackwell; 2011, p. 77–137.

7 Matthews D, Beatty S, Dyson P, King L, Meston N, Pal A, et al. *Diabetes: The Facts*. Oxford: Oxford University Press; 2008.

8 Haffner SM, Lehto S, Rönnemaa T, Pyörälä K, Laakso M. Mortality from coronary heart disease in subjects with type 2 diabetes and in nondiabetic subjects with and without prior myocardial infarction. *New England Journal of Medicine*. 1998; **339**(4): 229–34.

9 Donahoe SM, Stewart GC, McCabe CH, Mohanavelu S, Murphy SA, Cannon CP, et al. Diabetes and mortality following acute coronary syndromes. *Journal of the American Medical Association*. 2007; **298**(7): 765–75.

10 Malavige LS, Levy JC. Erectile dysfunction in diabetes mellitus. *Journal of Sexual Medicine*. 2009; **6**(5): 1232–47.

11 Singh N, Armstrong DG, Lipsky BA. Preventing foot ulcers in patients with diabetes. *Journal of the American Medical Association*. 2005; **293**(2): 217–28.

12 Daousi C, MacFarlane IA, Woodward A, Nurmikko TJ, Bundred PE,

Benbow SJ. Chronic painful peripheral neuropathy in an urban community: a controlled comparison of people with and without diabetes. *Diabetic Medicine.* 2004; **21**(9): 976–82.

13 Veves A, Backonja M, Malik RA. Painful diabetic neuropathy: epidemiology, natural history, early diagnosis, and treatment options. *Pain Medicine.* 2008; **9**(6): 660–74.

14 Vamos EP, Bottle A, Majeed A, Millett C. Trends in lower extremity amputations in people with and without diabetes in England, 1996–2005. *Diabetes Research and Clinical Practice.* 2010; **87**(2): 275–82.

15 Gale L, Vedhara K, Searle A, Kemple T, Campbell R. Patients' perspectives on foot complications in type 2 diabetes: a qualitative study. *British Journal of General Practice.* 2008; **58**(553): 555–63.

16 Morris D. Prevention and treatment of diabetic retinopathy. *Nurse Prescribing.* 2012; **12**(1): 22–4.

17 Berge LI, Riize T, Fasmer OB, Lund A, Oedegaard KJ, Hundal Ø. Risk of depression in diabetes is highest for young persons using oral anti-diabetic agents. *Diabetic Medicine.* 2012; **29**(4): 509–14.

5 Treating diabetes with drugs

1 Rosenfeld L. Insulin: discovery and controversy. *Clinical Chemistry.* 2002; **48**(12): 2270–88.

2 Matthews D, Beatty S, Dyson P, King L, Meston N, Pal A, et al. *Diabetes: The Facts.* Oxford: Oxford University Press; 2008.

3 Wright A, Burden AC, Paizey RB, Cull CA, Holman RR. Sulfonylurea inadequacy: efficacy of addition of insulin over 6 years in patients with type 2 diabetes in the UK. Prospective Diabetes Study (UKPDS 57). *Diabetes Care.* 2002; **25**(2): 330–6.

4 Tattersall R. *Diabetes: The Biography.* Oxford: Oxford University Press; 2009.

5 Mazze RS, Strock ES, Bergenstal RM, Criego A, Cuddihy R, Langer O, et al. Detection and treatment of type 1 diabetes. In: *Staged Diabetes Management.* Wiley-Blackwell; 2011, p. 41–75.

6 Furman BL. The development of Byetta (exenatide) from the venom of the Gila monster as an anti-diabetic agent. *Toxicon.* 2012; **9**(4): 464–71.

6 Treating diabetes by changing your lifestyle

1 Toeller M. Lifestyle Issues: Diet. In: *Textbook of Diabetes*. Wiley-Blackwell; 2010, p. 346–57.
2 Hamson K. Optimizing insulin therapy to individual need in type 2 diabetes. *Practice Nursing*. 2012; **23**(1): 33–6.
3 Matthews D, Beatty S, Dyson P, King L, Meston N, Pal A, et al. *Diabetes: The Facts*. Oxford: Oxford University Press; 2008.

7 Diet and diabetes – the first steps

1 Hoidrup S, Andreasen AH, Osler M, Pedersen AN, Jorgensen LM, Jorgensen T, et al. Assessment of habitual energy and macronutrient intake in adults: comparison of a seven day food record with a dietary history interview. *European Journal of Clinical Nutrition*. 2002; **56**(2): 105–13.

8 Controlling carbs

1 Toeller M. Lifestyle Issues: Diet. In: *Textbook of Diabetes*. Wiley-Blackwell; 2010, p. 346–57.
2 Atkinson FS, Foster-Powell K, Brand-Miller JC. International tables of glycemic index and glycemic load values: 2008. *Diabetes Care*. 2008; **31**(12): 2281–3.
3 Matthews D, Beatty S, Dyson P, King L, Meston N, Pal A, et al. *Diabetes: The Facts*. Oxford: Oxford University Press; 2008.

9 Diet and diabetes – beyond carbs

1 Matthews D, Beatty S, Dyson P, King L, Meston N, Pal A, et al. *Diabetes: The Facts*. Oxford: Oxford University Press; 2008.
2 Toeller M. Lifestyle Issues: Diet. In: *Textbook of Diabetes*. Wiley-Blackwell; 2010, p. 346–57.
3 Kromhout D, Yasuda S, Geleijnse JM, Shimokawa H. Fish oil and omega-3 fatty acids in cardiovascular disease: do they really work? *European Heart Journal*. 2012; **33**(4): 436–43.
4 Yokoyama M, Origasa H, Matsuzaki M, Matsuzawa Y, Saito Y, Ishikawa Y, et al. Effects of eicosapentaenoic acid on major coronary events in hypercholesterolaemic patients (JELIS): a randomized open-label, blinded end point analysis. *Lancet*. 2007; **369**(9567): 1090–8.

5 Yee P, Weymouth AE, Fletcher EL, Vingrys AJ. A role for omega-3 polyunsaturated fatty acid supplements in diabetic neuropathy. *Investigative Ophthalmology and Visual Science.* 2010; **51**(3): 1755–64.

6 Anderson JW, Conley SB. Whole Grains and Diabetes. *Whole Grains and Health.* Blackwell Publishing Professional; 2007, p. 29–46.

7 Hunter D, Foster M, McArthur JO, Ojha R, Petocz P, Samman S. Evaluation of the micronutrient composition of plant foods produced by organic and conventional agricultural methods. *Critical Reviews in Food Science and Nutrition.* 2011; **51**(6): 571–82.

8 Mazze RS, Strock ES, Bergenstal RM, Criego A, Cuddihy R, Langer O, et al. Detection and treatment of type 1 diabetes. In: *Staged Diabetes Management.* Wiley-Blackwell; 2011, p. 41–75.

9 Toeller M. Lifestyle Issues: Diet. In: *Textbook of Diabetes.* Wiley-Blackwell; 2010, p. 346–57.

10 Using supplements safely

1 Baquer NZ, Kumar P, Taha A, Kale RK, Cowsik SM, McLean P. Metabolic and molecular action of *Trigonella foenum-graecum* (fenugreek) and trace metals in experimental diabetic tissues. *Journal of Biosciences.* 2011; **36**(2): 383–96.

2 Toeller M. Lifestyle Issues: Diet. In: *Textbook of Diabetes.* Wiley-Blackwell; 2010, p. 346–57.

3 Halat KM, Dennehy CE. Botanicals and dietary supplements in diabetic peripheral neuropathy. *Journal of the American Board of Family Practice.* 2003; **16**(1): 47–57.

4 Golbidi S, Badran M, Laher I. Diabetes and alpha lipoic acid. *Frontiers in Pharmacology.* 2011; **2**: 69.

5 Bolland MJ, Avenell A, Baron JA, Grey A, MacLennan GS, Gamble GD, et al. Effect of calcium supplements on risk of myocardial infarction and cardiovascular events: meta-analysis. *BMJ.* 2010; 341: c3691.

6 Anderson JW, Conley SB. Whole Grains and Diabetes. *Whole Grains and Health.* Blackwell Publishing Professional; 2007, p. 29–46.

7 Sun Y, Lai MS, Lu CJ. Effectiveness of vitamin B_{12} on diabetic neuropathy: systematic review of clinical controlled trials. *Acta Neurologica Taiwanica.* 2005; **14**(2): 48–54.

8 Vinik AI, Maser RE, Mitchell BD, Freeman R. Diabetic autonomic neuropathy. *Diabetes Care.* 2003; **26**(5): 1553–79.

9 Shim JE, Paik HY, Shin CS, Park KS, Lee HK. Vitamin C nutriture in newly diagnosed diabetes. *Journal of Nutritional Science and Vitaminology.* 2010; **56**(4): 217–21.

10 Will JC, Byers T. Does diabetes mellitus increase the requirement for vitamin C? *Nutrition Reviews.* 1996; **54**(7): 193–202.

11 Renneberg R. Biotech history: yew trees, paclitaxel synthesis and fungi. *Biotechnology Journal.* 2007; **2**(10): 1207–9.

12 Tattersall R. *Diabetes: The Biography.* Oxford: Oxford University Press; 2009.

13 Leung L, Birtwhistle R, Kotecha J, Hannah S, Cuthbertson S. Anti-diabetic and hypoglycaemic effects of *Momordica charantia* (bitter melon): a mini review. *British Journal of Nutrition.* 2009; **102**(12): 1703–8.

14 Jia L, Zhao Y, Liang XJ. Current evaluation of the millennium phytomedicine–ginseng (II): Collected chemical entities, modern pharmacology, and clinical applications emanated from traditional Chinese medicine. *Current Medicinal Chemistry.* 2009; **16**(22): 2924–42.

15 Hahm SW, Park J, Son YS. *Opuntia humifusa* stems lower blood glucose and cholesterol levels in streptozotocin-induced diabetic rats. *Nutrition Research.* 2011; **31**(6): 479–87.

11 Putting it all together

1 Matthews D, Beatty S, Dyson P, King L, Meston N, Pal A, et al. *Diabetes: The Facts.* Oxford: Oxford University Press; 2008.

Further reading

Christine Craggs-Hinton, Adam Balen, *Coping with Polycystic Ovary Syndrome*. London: Sheldon Press; 2008.

Susan Elliot-Wright, *Coping with Type 2 Diabetes*. London: Sheldon Press; 2006.

Sander L. Gilman, *Obesity: The Biography*. Oxford: Oxford University Press; 2010.

Mark Greener, *The Heart Attack Survival Guide*. London: Sheldon Press; 2012.

David Matthews, Sue Beatty, Pam Dyson, Laurie King, Niki Meston, Aparna Pal et al., *Diabetes: The Facts*. Oxford: Oxford University Press; 2008.

Tom Smith, *Living with Type 1 Diabetes*. London: Sheldon Press; 2010.

Robert Tattersall, *Diabetes: The Biography*. Oxford: Oxford University Press; 2009.

Index